THE
14-DAY
NO
SUGAR
DIET

D0932201

GALVAN!ZED
Books

This book proposes a program of diet and exercise recommendations for the reader to follow. However, you should consult a qualified medical professional (and, if you are pregnant, your ob-gyn) before starting this or any other diet or fitness program. Please seek your doctor's advice before making any decisions that affect your health or extreme changes in your diet, particularly if you suffer from any medical condition or have any symptom that may require treatment. As with any diet or exercise program, if at any time you experience discomfort, stop immediately and consult your physician.

Mention of specific companies, organizations, or authorities in this book does not imply endorsement by the author or publisher, nor does mention of specific companies, organizations, or authorities imply that they endorse this book, its author, or the publisher.

Design by Andy Turnbull

THE
14-DAY
NO
SUGAR
DIET

LOSE UP TO A
POUND A DAY
AND FIND YOUR PATH
TO BETTER HEALTH

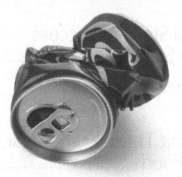

BY *NEW YORK TIMES* BESTSELLING AUTHOR
JEFF CSATARI
AND THE EDITORS OF *EAT THIS, NOT THAT!*

Contents

THE
14-DAY
NO
SUGAR
DIET

INTRODUCTION

Sugar Scare

A **SIMPLE BLOOD TEST** changed my life. It may have even saved my life because the results revealed something about me that I didn't know and would never have guessed: I had a problem with sugar.

My doctor told me I had "prediabetes." A prediabetes diagnosis meant my blood sugar level was higher than it should be but not yet high enough to be classified as "type

2 diabetes." Prediabetes is one key condition in a cluster of health problems (including high blood pressure, abnormal cholesterol, and a high triglyceride level) that some doctors refer to as "metabolic syndrome." This cluster of health issues increases my risk of heart disease and stroke. The blood test showed that I could be on the express train headed for full-blown type 2 diabetes and could potentially need daily insulin injections if I didn't make some lifestyle changes to prevent it from getting worse.

This was all a huge shock to me. Actually, I left my doctor's office shaking. See, as a health journalist for nearly two decades, I've been well aware of prediabetes and the frightening things that can happen if it turns into type 2 diabetes and isn't managed properly. Having high levels of glucose (sugar) in your blood means your body isn't processing the sugar you get from foods properly to use as energy. Untreated, elevated blood sugar can damage your heart, brain, kidneys, and eyes. Diabetes can lead to limb amputation, blindness, kidney, and nerve damage, and Alzheimer's disease. So, you can imagine why this news worried me. And why it surprised me. I had no idea I was getting too much sugar in my diet.

You might not either.

But that's exactly why diabetes should concern you, too. It can sneak up on you even when you think your health is fine. This book will show you where to find the sources of hidden sugars in your diet and how to reduce their negative impact on your health. The good news for all of us is that by taking control of our health with the simple steps outlined in this book we can drop pounds, lose belly fat (a key risk factor for diabetes), and keep our blood sugar under control all at the same time. And if you have prediabetes or even type 2 diabetes, you can reverse that diagnosis, doctors say, through simple changes to your eating habits and getting more physical activity every day. It worked for me and I know it can work for you, too.

Your No Sugar Solution

Type 2 diabetes is a dangerous disease that is now reaching epidemic proportions in the United States and most of the world. From 1988 to 2014, the number of people with the disease has increased by 382 percent. Now, nearly 10 percent of the U.S. population, or 29 million people, have diabetes, according to the American Diabetes Association, and more than a quarter don't know they have it. Many, many more Americans are headed toward a type 2 diagnosis. The Centers for Disease Control and Prevention (CDC) says 86 percent of adult Americans—that's more than a third of the population—are living with *prediabetes*. The CDC says 90 percent of them have no idea they are at risk.

How the heck did I become one of them? I write about nutrition and exercise every day. I believed my diet was much healthier than that of most people simply because I'm exposed to nutrition information every day. It's my job to keep up with medical journals with names like *Clinical Nutrition, Journal of Endocrinology,* and *JAMA, The Journal of the American Medical Association.* I'm a runner. I lift weights pretty regularly. I'm not obese. I rarely drink soda. I don't smoke. And because of all of the above, I never thought to have my blood sugar level tested. Ever.

Then, while doing research for a book about healthy aging, I went to Quest Diagnostics for a blood draw to test for various markers of health, including high blood sugar. The test that revealed my prediabetes is called the hemoglobin A1c blood test (HbA1c for short). Hemoglobin (Hb) is a protein in red blood cells that carries oxygen from the lungs to the body's tissues. When a person's blood sugar becomes high, glucose (a type of sugar) attaches to the hemoglobin. The hemoglobin becomes *glycosylated*. Think of a jelly doughnut (the red blood cell) covered in powdered sugar (the glucose). The glucose stays attached for the life of the red blood cells, about 2 to 3 months. So a HbA1c test measures the amount of sugarcoated hemoglobin in the blood for several months before the test. That's what makes the test so useful; it measures high blood sugar over time.

My HbA1c topped 5.8 percent, which put me in the prediabetes category, according to my doctor, Florence Comite, MD, an endocrinologist in New York City. Now, some doctors wouldn't be very alarmed at my score. It's on the low end of the prediabetes spectrum, but Dr. Comite is more aggressive than most. She practices what's called Precision Medicine, looking deep into one's whole physiology to prevent disease before it emerges. She knew that I had a family history of diabetes, so she wanted to make sure I nipped this in the bud. And subsequent blood tests suggested that my numbers were trending toward diabetes. If your HbA1c results are 6.5 percent or higher, you have type 2 diabetes. Now that I think about it, I should have been smarter about getting checked out sooner. My mom has had elevated blood sugar over the years. And my grandfather was diabetic.

Your Crystal Ball

HbA1c is one of the most useful diagnostic tests and predictors of your potential longevity. It's like peering into a crystal ball to see your health future. How? Because the higher your numbers, the higher your chances for developing long-term health problems caused by consistently elevated blood sugar levels. Your blood sugar has a huge impact on your veins and tissues and can, over time, trigger a host of problems including obesity, heart attacks, strokes, kidney failure, vision problems, and numbness in your legs or feet. That's scary stuff.

But that scary stuff doesn't happen overnight, or even next month, which, for some people, makes doing anything about their high blood sugar seem less urgent. But while kidney failure may not be in *your* near future, consider something that your high blood sugar could be doing to you right now: storing belly fat. The carbohydrates that you eat, especially those simple sugars like high fructose corn syrup and others that are added to processed foods to make them taste sweet, are not benign; they impact your body in significant ways.

See, sugar causes your body to release the hormone insulin. And when insulin is present in your bloodstream, you don't burn body fat, you store it, typically in your abdomen and thighs. So, if you're looking for an urgent reason to pay attention to your blood sugar levels, and even if you aren't worried about your health five years from now, think about the upcoming beach season.

My hope, however, is that you'll be more concerned about the health impact of a continuous overload of sugar bombarding your body than just fitting into a swimsuit. Here's what's happening inside you that you can't see when you have high blood sugar: When you eat something high in carbohydrates and get a sugar-level spike or the sugar stays in your bloodstream too long, the insulin that has been deployed to clear it from your bloodstream can't work fast enough. The excess glucose (sugar) stays there and it becomes corrosive to your veins and tissues. To protect your tissues, your body has a backup plan: It converts and stores the sugar as fat. If your blood sugar spikes again and again and again from a regular diet of high-carbohydrate meals and sugary drinks, more and more insulin is needed to do the same job that a little did before. This is insulin resistance or what's commonly known as prediabetes. If nothing is done to reverse prediabetes, eventually your pancreas may stop producing insulin and you become diabetic. This is type 2 diabetes. You may need to take medication to help your body clear sugar from your bloodstream. If lifestyle changes and prescription pills do not manage the disease, you may need to inject synthetic insulin.

Losing just 7 percent of your body weight can cut your risk of developing diabetes by 60 percent.

Now you can understand why I was so concerned about my prediabetes diagnosis. I have a family. I want to be as healthy as possible for as long as possible. Fortunately, I have a proactive doctor and a lot of research material at my disposal. I took my diagnosis very seriously and started schooling myself on things that

I could do to reverse my prediabetes. The first and easiest step is something you can begin doing today: Spot the added sugars in your foods and start avoiding them.

As I mentioned earlier, the good news for me and you is that there is so much we can do on our own to bring our blood sugar under control. It starts with knowledge, says Michael Pinone, MD, MPH, who is a member of the U.S. Preventive Services Task Force that recently recommended screening for high blood glucose in all overweight adults 40 to 70 years of age. "If we can identify people at risk and help them make lifestyle changes, we may decrease their risk of progressing to diabetes, and prevent the serious complications associated with this illness," he says.

By following my doctor's advice and using the strategies in this book, I've reduced my HbA1c enough that I'm no longer prediabetic. Plus, I've lost 10 pounds of fat while adding 6 pounds of muscle. And I feel great. Now, I want you to enjoy the same health-altering results that I did by sharing these simple strategies with you.

Prediabetes and type 2 diabetes are serious health issues. If you suspect you have high blood sugar, ask your doctor to test you. If you're like I was and feel that you're in the clear, answer the self-check questions on page 18. Your results may give you the extra nudge you need to schedule a visit to your doctor to be properly evaluated. If you are already prediabetic or diabetic, carefully follow your doctor's treatment plan. It's critical that people who are taking insulin for diabetes do not stop therapy unless directed to do so by their physician. This book is not a substitute for medication or a doctor's treatment.

But you can use this book as additional firepower to build a fitter, healthier body right now and prevent this dangerous disease from ever giving you trouble. Build a plan using this book. Be realistic. You're not going to lower a high A1c overnight. It takes time. However, following the 14-Day No Sugar Diet plan will put you on the fast track to eating healthier for life, gaining control over your blood sugar, and losing pounds. I can't stress enough how important it is to lose weight. It's *the best thing* you can do to improve your health and prevent type 2 diabetes, and the benefits start occurring very quickly. Scientists at the American Diabetes Association cite studies proving that losing just 7 percent of your body weight can cut your risk of developing the disease by nearly 60 percent.

Think about that for a sec. If you weigh 160 pounds, that's about 11 pounds. You can lose that in two or three weeks. If you weigh 280 pounds, 7 percent is about 20 pounds. So, you can see how much you can personally impact your health without resorting to drugs. In just two weeks, you can build the foundation of a lifestyle to prevent a disease that targets just about everyone.

CHAPTER 1

Lose Weight, Live Longer

The benefits of the 14-Day No Sugar Diet

HERE'S THE wonderful news about starting a plan to reduce the amount of added sugars in your daily diet: It will have a snowball effect on your entire life. Everything you do to prevent the progression of prediabetes will help you look and feel better and perform at your best. Eating healthier will encourage you to be more active. You'll handle stress better, improve your sleep habits, and feel more optimistic about life. Everybody wants those things and everyone can have them by making some simple daily changes that you'll find in this book. Here's exactly what you can expect to gain:

You'll Curb Cravings and Feel Fuller Longer

Nutrition researchers from the University of Copenhagen found that basing meals around high-fiber plant foods like those used in the 14-Day No Sugar Diet meal plan improved feelings of satiety. That means making a few simple adjustments to your dinner plate can keep you from succumbing to the call of cookies and ice cream an hour after supper. Study participants felt fuller longer than those who consumed meat protein meals. In fact, the subjects who ate protein from beans and peas consumed an average of 12 percent fewer calories at their next meal than if they had eaten meat. Think about that: Meals with meat are typically very satiating, but this study showed that high-fiber plant protein was even more effective at keeping post-meal cravings at bay.

You'll Improve Your Insulin Sensitivity

According to a double blind clinical study published in the *Journal of Nutrition* in 2010, obese, insulin-resistant people who drank two blueberry smoothies daily and did nothing else to change their lifestyles or diets boosted their insulin sensitivity by 10 percent or more. This is important because being resistant to insulin can lead to type 2 diabetes. (Check out chapter 8's delicious low-sugar smoothie recipes.) Remember, you want your body to be sensitive to insulin, so you can metabolize blood sugars more efficiently.

You'll Cut Your Risk of Developing Type 2 Diabetes in Half

Excess weight is the single most important cause of type 2 diabetes. In fact, being obese makes you up to 40 times more likely to develop diabetes than someone who is a normal weight. But by following the 14-Day No Sugar Diet, you should be able to safely lose enough weight to dramatically cut your risk. Remember what those diabetes scientists found? Losing just 7 percent of your body weight can cut your chances of developing type 2 diabetes by nearly 60 percent. Make that your goal. Even a 5 percent reduction in weight delivers significant benefits.

You'll Have More Energy

Fatigue is a common complaint of people who eat lots of sugars and have high blood sugar. But managing high blood sugar by limiting certain foods can cause exhaustion, too, because cells are being deprived of fuel. The balancing act needs to be done right. Our structured meal plan will help keep your blood sugar stable while maintaining a high energy level throughout the day so you won't need caffeine or chocolate pick-me-ups to get you through the doldrums.

You'll Strengthen Your Muscles

Every time you see a sugar bowl, a box of sugary cereal, or a bottle of juice containing HFCS (high fructose corn syrup), I want you to think "muscle shrinker" because that's what sugar is. Scientists have recently linked refined sugar intake to age-related muscle wasting, a condition that doctors call *sarcopenia*. After age 30, your muscle mass and strength naturally start to decline. A poor diet full of sugary, processed foods can speed up the progression of sarcopenia. And muscle loss can speed up the progression from prediabetes to type 2 diabetes. Do you see how diet impacts muscle and muscle impacts your health? You truly are what you eat! Recent research by scientists from the University of Delaware and the National Institute on Aging suggests that reducing starchy, sweet, and processed foods may help us hold on to our precious muscle and strength. And when you have more muscle mass, uptake of glucose improves, reducing your risk of insulin resistance.

You'll Improve Your Heart Health

A 2012 study by Johns Hopkins Medical School researchers showed that a diet that's low in carbohydrates could improve artery function. Also that year, an analysis of 23 clinical studies published in the *American Journal of Epidemiology* found that keeping blood sugar stable with a low-carbohydrate diet is effective at reducing risk of metabolic syndrome and heart disease. Compared to people on a low-fat diet, low-carb eaters in this study significantly reduced their total cholesterol, LDL (bad) cholesterol and triglyceride levels and improved their HDL (good) cholesterol. The 14-Day No Sugar Diet will dramatically reduce your reliance on high-carb processed foods that lead to heart problems.

Your Belly Will Shrink

Carrying a big belly is the number 1 risk factor for type 2 diabetes. Fortunately, there's a well-documented remedy for too much belly fat: a reduced-sugar diet. By changing your habit of eating high-calorie sugary carbs, your body will respond by burning fat stored around your middle for energy instead of all those sugars from processed carbs. Researchers compared losing weight through a low-fat diet and a low-carb diet in subjects over the course of a six-month diet plan. Each test group ate the same number of calories in their diets; only the carb and fat content differed. It turned out that the low-carb dieters lost an average of 10 pounds more than those on the low-fat diet. What's more, the researchers found that belly fat loss percentage was much higher for the low-carb group than the low-fat group.

You'll Feel Happier

By shrinking your belly fat, you'll reduce levels of the stress hormone cortisol that's associated with a buildup of visceral fat, the dangerous fat that surrounds your organs. In the Study of Women's Health Across the Nation, researchers found that middle-aged women who had more visceral belly fat also had more hostility and symptoms of depression. According to a different study of 12,000 people by researchers at the University of Warwick, improving the diet by adding more servings of fruits and vegetables incrementally improves feelings of happiness. Most dramatically, people who went from eating almost no produce to eight daily portions of fruits and vegetables boosted their psychological well-being as much as they would if they went from being unemployed to employed.

You'll Think Clearer

Avoiding the sugar crush can also do wonders for keeping you as smart as a whip, suggests new research exploring the impact of food on the brain. Reduced levels of insulin in the blood and markers of inflammation correlated with improved cognitive function, especially memory, in a study at the University of Münster. Researchers there placed subjects between ages 50 and 80 into one of three groups. One group ate a lower-calorie diet, one group a diet low in saturated fat, and the third ate as they normally did. At the end of the 3-month experiment, only the low-calorie group experienced a significant (above 20 percent) improvement in their ability to recall words on a list. That clear-thinking group also had the lowest blood insulin and lowest levels of an inflammation marker called C-reactive protein.

You'll Protect Yourself from Dementia

Several studies, including research published in the *New England Journal of Medicine,* have linked high blood sugar to dementia. In fact, some doctors refer to Alzheimer's disease as "type 3 diabetes." Why? Well, insulin is a vasodilator that increases blood flow throughout the body, including the brain. When you have insulin resistance, cerebral blood flow is compromised. Poor blood flow affects neuroplasticity, or brain plasticity, the brain's amazing ability to change and adapt by forming new connections between neurons.

CHAPTER 2

Start Shedding Sugar Pounds Now

Get a head start in four simple steps

BEFORE YOU embark on the 14-Day No Sugar Diet program, I'd like you to do something. You can start it now even before you read beyond this chapter. Call it a warm-up or pre-game prep.

Maybe you played a sport or an instrument in high school. Before any competition or performance, and even before every practice session, you probably went through a ritual of stretching, warm-up exercises, drills, and visualization to get ready. Remember? There's a simple reason every athlete, musician, or actor does this: A physically and mentally warmed-up body performs better and is more successful.

So, doing this easy head start below will help you begin to minimize sugar's impact on your body and lose more weight quicker once you start the 14-Day No Sugar Diet plan that's detailed a little later in the book. These are just four simple steps, but they will make it so much easier, mentally and physically, to adopt the lifestyle changes of the program.

You'll gain four powerful benefits from this head start:

• you'll eliminate mindless snacking;

• you'll block the pervasive cravings that often sabotage healthy eating habits;

• you'll cut sugary liquid calories from your diet, which is one of the quickest ways to drop significant pounds;

• you'll understand how sugary carbs affect your body. And that will give you an enormous advantage for striking a sugar balance.

Begin this program with momentum. Here are four steps to give you a head start:

Step 1

Identify the Hidden Calories

It's easy to ignore the number of calories in a beverage. Liquid goes down so effortlessly. You don't have to chew. And it doesn't really fill you up so it's hard to remember how much you've had. This exercise will help: Grab an index card and a pen. Keep them in your pocket all day. Whenever you drink something—from water to wine and everything liquid in between—write down what you had and how much. At the end of the day, look at your drink list. If you're like most Americans, there's not much pure water on your list but a lot of high-calorie drinks, especially sugar-sweetened beverages. Now, for a real surprise, tally up the number of liquid calories you consumed in that one day. And remember, a bottle of juice or soda often contains two or more servings. So, be sure to get the math right if you drank the whole bottle. What did you get? How many calories came from drink? How many carbs? How many grams of sugar from beverages did you consume that day? Eye-opening, isn't it?

Step 2

Substitute Water for Sweet Drinks

Soft drinks account for 33 percent of our total intake of added sweeteners. Depending on which study you read, it's estimated that the average American adult swallows between 150 and 400 beverage calories a day. Some folks drink a lot more. How does your liquid list compare?

Liquid calories—soda, 100-percent fruit juice, fruit punch, milk, sweetened coffee and tea—are easy to miss because they go down so quickly and easily and they typically don't fill you up. Because they are such a big part of your calories—easily 20 percent of your daily calorie intake —evaporating those calories is the best way for you to lose significant pounds and beat diabetes.

How to do it? You guessed it: Drink water. There's no better beverage for good health. In a French study, researchers found that drinking four or more 8-ounce glasses of water likely protects against high blood sugar, the precursor to metabolic syndrome and type 2 diabetes. The study involving 3,615 men and women showed that those who reported drinking more than 34 ounces of water a day were 21 percent less likely to develop high blood sugar over the next nine years than those who drank 16 or fewer ounces daily.

Step 3

Put a Dent in Mindless Eating

One day, I saw a bowl of potato chips on the kitchen counter. My daughter had brought it up from the basement where she was watching TV with some friends. Each time I walked past the bowl, I dipped my hand in. On the fourth or fifth pass, I took a paper towel and put a pile of chips on it to take into my office.

I must have eaten half a bag without even thinking about it.

That's a perfect example of mindless snacking. How often do you do that? Most of us don't remember many of the foods we consume because we snack automatically when we see something salty or sweet within arm's reach. It doesn't even register.

If you're trying to resist temptation, a bowl of salt and vinegar potato chips within easy reach is not the way to do it. You know that. But researchers at Cornell University and the University of Illinois wanted to prove it, scientifically. In an experiment, they placed dishes of chocolate candies in an office setting in different locations that made the chocolate either easy to see and reach or not very visible or convenient to grab. They found that when the candy dishes were easy to see and convenient to reach, office workers ate 5.6 more chocolates per day than when the dishes were visible but inconvenient to access and 2.9 more candies when the dishes were convenient but not visible. What this means to you: Hide those high-calorie snacks. Make them hard to see and access at the back of a pantry shelf. Instead, keep a bowl of fruit or cut-up vegetables front and center on the kitchen counter. You're more likely to snack on the good stuff if it's staring you in the face.

Step 4

Write "Low Sugar/High Fiber" on the Top of Your Grocery List

Next time you make out your grocery shopping list, write "Low Sugar/High Fiber" on top and review what you're planning to buy while keeping those four words in mind. Then revise your list. Erase most of the groceries that don't fit under one of those categories. Doing that should automatically steer your grocery cart toward the perimeter of the store where you'll find the whole foods: fresh produce, dairy, eggs, fresh meats, poultry, and fish. Here's why this is a key practice:

It's well documented that a diet rich in processed foods, low-quality carbohydrates, and other foods that cause spikes in blood sugar can lead to type 2 diabetes. And guess what? Processed foods, low-quality carbs, and other foods that trigger blood sugar spikes make up the bulk of the typical American grocery cart. A recent study in the *American Journal of Clinical Nutrition* analyzed grocery shopping habits of 157,142 households and found that 61 percent of food purchased came from highly processed foods and beverages, in other words, packaged foods that are loaded with saturated fat, sugar, and lots of preservatives to ensure long shelf life. Sixty-one percent! If you add in moderately processed foods, then more than 75 percent of all the energy we consume comes from a box, bag, jar, or can. Get in the habit of eating fresh and clean.

Head Start Summary

Step 1. Identify Hidden Calories

Step 2. Substitute Water for Sweet Drinks

Step 3. Put a Dent in Mindless Eating

Step 4. Write "Low Sugar/High Fiber" on the Top of Your Grocery List

CHAPTER 3

How Sugar Trouble Starts

To prevent high blood sugar, know the enemy and how it attacks

I REMEMBER MY grandfather poking his swollen feet with the end of his cane. He said they felt numb.

"I have sugar," he explained.

At 8 years old, I didn't understand. Sugar was the stuff in the bowl that we had just sprinkled on our blintzes. I didn't know he was referring to "adult-onset diabetes," which is what type 2 diabetes was known as back in the late 1960s. My family just called it "having sugar."

Type 2 "sugar" didn't show up in Grandpop until his 80s. He was lean and active all his life—a coal miner and a laborer in a brick factory—but age is a risk factor for problems with sugar. So is high blood pressure, which he had. This is important to know because having a family history of type 2 diabetes makes you more susceptible to the disease.

As I've said before, type 2 diabetes doesn't invade your body overnight. It's a long-term process that can sneak up on you. But it's occurring at younger and younger ages. Even children are now developing type 2 diabetes.

Knowledge is your first line of defense. By knowing the risk factors and understanding how high blood sugar happens in your body and develops into diabetes, you can take action long before a doctor needs to get involved.

Type 2 Diabetes Risk Factors

You are more likely to develop prediabetes and type 2 diabetes if...

- you are age 45 or older
- you are overweight or obese
- you have excess abdominal fat or a large waist
- you aren't physically active
- you have a family history of diabetes
- you have high blood pressure
- you have a history of gestational diabetes
- you are African American, American Indian, Asian American, Hispanic/Latino
- you have a history of heart disease or stroke
- you suffer from depression

As you can gather from the risk factors above, there are some things, like your age and heritage, that you can't do anything about. But just look at what you can control: your weight through the foods you eat and moving your body more, the two factors that prevent type 2 diabetes best!

Know Your Carbs

Do you know about the three macronutrients? They are protein, fat, and carbohydrates. Protein and fat do not raise blood sugar. Carbohydrates do, so let's focus on carbs because there seems to be a lot of confusion around this macronutrient.

Carbohydrates are made up of sugars, starches, and fiber. They are found in all kinds of healthy and unhealthy foods, from bread, pasta, and milk to fruits and vegetables, soda, and apple pie. Reducing your consumption of carbs can help you manage your blood sugar, but paying attention to carbohydrate *quality* is more important than carbohydrate *quantity*. Here's why:

When you eat any kind of carbohydrate, digestion breaks the food down into glucose (blood sugar), the fuel that powers your body and brain. But unhealthy carbs enter the bloodstream very quickly, and that's what causes unhealthy spikes in blood sugar.

Unhealthy, easily-digested carbohydrates are usually highly processed or refined foods like soda, white bread, pastries, fruit drinks, and sweeteners like table sugar, honey, maple syrup, and corn syrup. Those sweeteners are used in lots of baked goods and packaged foods, too.

The healthiest carbohydrates include unprocessed or minimally processed whole grains, vegetables, beans, and fruits. We call these carbs the healthy ones because they are typically high in fiber content, they digest more slowly and, therefore, deliver a more gradual impact on your blood sugar. Plus, they contain lots of important vitamins and minerals that you don't typically get from, say, a chocolate glazed doughnut.

Why is the speed that sugar enters the bloodstream so important? It has to do with what happens next. When your blood receives glucose, your pancreas notices and responds by secreting the hormone insulin into your bloodstream. If your blood gets a huge jolt of sugar because you just had two glasses of wine (or sweet tea) with your spaghetti dinner, your pancreas sends more insulin to deal with the overload of glucose.

Insulin acts like a key to unlock cells and allow glucose to enter and be used for energy. Insulin helps store excess sugar that doesn't make it into the cells in the liver where it can be used when blood sugar levels dip. Insulin helps keep blood sugar balanced. Most of the time, that is.

If your diet is full of fast-absorbed sugars from sweets, sodas, juices, pasta, French fries, rice, and baked goods, the wild swings in blood sugar eventually cause your cells to become numb or resistant to the insulin and they won't take the sugar in. Your pancreas responds by sending more insulin to balance your blood sugar. This is what's known as insulin resistance.

Over time, your cells become so resistant to the insulin that too much sugar remains left in your bloodstream and your pancreas can't pump out enough insulin to do the job. And your doctor may diagnose you as diabetic.

Now you are at risk for prolonged high blood sugar's corrosive effects on blood vessels. In addition, all that ineffective insulin in your blood starts to tell your body to store fat around your belly area, setting you up for a myriad of

Type 1 vs Type 2

Type 1 *diabetes mellitus* is an autoimmune condition that results in the pancreas producing little or no insulin. There is no cure.

Type 2 *diabetes mellitus* is a chronic condition caused by a combination of genetics and lifestyle factors that results in high blood sugar from insulin resistance. Type 2 diabetes can be managed through weight loss, controlling carbohydrates, physical activity, and medication. It is possible to reverse symptoms to regain health.

---

health problems including stiffening of the arteries and high blood pressure, high cholesterol, high triglycerides, and inflammation.

Sorry, if that all seems scary. There's no way to sugar-coat the dangers of high blood sugar. However, by knowing how the foods you choose affect your diabetes risk, you can use your brain and body to protect yourself.

At the risk of sounding like a song on repeat, the good news is that type 2 diabetes can be prevented, even reversed. If you transform your body by eliminating added sugars, eating healthy whole foods, getting regular physical activity, and losing weight, you won't need a doctor to treat diabetes. Because there will be no diabetes to treat.

Could You Have Prediabetes?

Prediabetes means your blood sugar is higher than normal, but not yet high enough to officially be type 2 diabetes. Find out your risk for prediabetes by taking this simple self-test.*

Answer these seven questions. For each "yes" answer, record the number of points listed. "No" answers score 0 points.

YES	NO	
1	0	1. Are you a woman who has had a baby weighing more than 9 pounds at birth?
1	0	2. Do you have a sister or brother with diabetes?
1	0	3. Do you have a parent with diabetes?
5	0	4. Find your height on the "At-Risk Weight Chart" on the next page. Do you weigh as much as or more than the weight listed for your height?
5	0	5. Are you younger than 65 and get little or no exercise in a typical day?
5	0	6. Are you between ages 45 and 64?
9	0	7. Are you age 65 or older?

Add your score and check it against the score key.

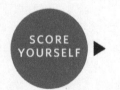

SCORE YOURSELF ▶

3 TO 8 POINTS means...
Your risk is likely to be currently low for having prediabetes.

9 POINTS OR MORE means...
Your risk is high for having prediabetes. See your family doctor and ask to be tested for high blood sugar.

At-Risk Weight Chart

Height	Weight (lbs.)	Height	Weight (lbs.)
4'10"	129	5'7"	172
4'11"	133	5'8"	177
5'0"	138	5'9"	182
5'1"	143	5'10"	188
5'2"	147	5'11"	193
5'3"	152	6'0"	199
5'4"	157	6'1"	204
5'5"	162	6'2"	210
5'6"	167	6'3"	216
		6'4"	221

* Adapted from the CDC National Diabetes Prevention Program

Know Your Numbers
Ask your doctor to test your blood sugar

◼ Don't wait for your doctor to suggest a test for diabetes. Ask for one to know where you stand. The American Diabetes Association recommends blood glucose screening starting at age 45 or sooner if you are overweight and have a family history of type 2 diabetes.

There are three blood tests your doctor may use to diagnose prediabetes or diabetes:

HbA1c (glycated hemoglobin) — This test measures blood sugar levels over 2 to 3 months by checking the percentage of red blood cells (hemoglobin) with sugar attached. Fasting isn't required. Blood is drawn through a vein at a lab or finger stick in your doctor's office or with a home kit.

Fasting blood sugar test — Measures blood sugar level from a blood sample taken after an overnight or 8-hour fast.

Oral glucose tolerance test — Most often used to diagnose gestational diabetes during pregnancy. A blood sample is taken after an overnight fast. Then you'll drink a very sweet solution and have your blood sugar level sampled again after two hours to determine how effectively insulin ushers the glucose out of your bloodstream.

What the Test Numbers Mean

	HbA1c	Fasting Blood Sugar	Oral Glucose Tolerance
Diabetes	6.5% or above	126 mg/dL or above	200 mg/dL or above
Prediabetes	5.7% to 6.4%	100 mg/dL to 125	140 mg/dL to 199
Normal	About 5	99 mg/dL or below	139 mg/dL or below

Source: Adapted from American Diabetes Association

CHAPTER

4

Six Powerful Steps to Success with the No Sugar Diet

How to use this plan to strip away 14 pounds and dramatically improve your health in just 14 days

THE 14-DAY No Sugar Diet can put you on the fast track to cutting your reliance on sweets and preventing one of the most preventable of diseases. The important thing to realize is that YOU are in control of your health future.

You have the amazing ability to transform your life and be healthier, leaner, fitter, and happier by being mindful of what you eat and moving your body more. Moving more and thinking twice before you bring that spoon, fork, or glass to your lips. You can do that. You're going to see what you're capable of, and that's going to give you the confidence to change your life with this 2-week plan. And it's highly likely that quick success is going to motivate you to keep going, to continue to make the long-term lifestyle changes you need to put the risk of diabetes to rest.

Science has proven that you have what it takes: Dozens of clinical studies have shown a direct correlation between losing a very achievable amount of your body weight—just 5 to 7 percent!—and slashing your type 2 diabetes risk significantly. If you're a 185-pound woman, 5 percent is less than 10 pounds away from significantly improving your health.

Do you see how empowering that truth can be? It means YOU, not your doctor, not the pharmaceutical industry, but *you* are in charge here. You don't have to fall prey to high blood sugar. You can beat type 2 diabetes.

I believe in you. *You* just need to believe in you. Together, we are going to fight high blood sugar with a six-step plan that will help you achieve three main goals:

A) **Slash the added sugars** mostly by overcoming your addiction to sweet treats and beverages and avoiding processed foods loaded with hidden sugars.

B) **Lose 5 to 7 percent of your body weight** by adopting a healthier eating style that you'll be able enjoy for the rest of your life.

C) **Get off the couch.** Move more every day. You don't even have to use the word "exercise." Find something active that's fun and makes you want to get off those sofa cushions. It will become addictive.

In the previous pages, you've read about the dangers of chronic high blood sugar and how type 2 diabetes happens. So, now you know why these are our three key goals.

When you cut added sugars from your diet, you automatically lose body fat. When you carry less body fat, your body manages blood sugar better. When you move your muscles, your body makes more efficient use of the glucose, the sugar fuel from foods—and your blood sugar stays stable.

Now, that sounds logical, even simple. But you probably know from previous attempts to drop pounds and get back in shape that it can be easier said than done. I hear you. I've been there. But I know that a systematic approach that's reasonable, and that doesn't require big, uncomfortable changes and painful sacrifices, will yield results for you that last.

Let's get into the nitty-gritty of the No Sugar Diet plan that will help you lose weight and put you on the right track toward much improved health over the next 14 days.

The 14-Day No Sugar Diet at

Step 1

Determine Your Goal Weight

Calculate the number of pounds to lose to cut your diabetes risk in half. Research has determined that it's as little as 5 percent to 7 percent. (See page 26 for details.) Make that your goal. You can do it! The next 5 steps will help to get you there.

Step 2

Eat Breakfast, Eat When You're Hungry, Eat Simply

By changing your relationship with food using some simple strategies, you'll keep your blood sugar stable and avoid cravings and bingeing. Don't worry, you'll still enjoy what you eat. Lose weight by following the No Sugar Diet Meal Plan, which incorporates delicious proteins and healthy carbohydrates.

Step 3

Banish Those Sneaky Sugar Sources

Know your enemies and keep them out of your mouth. You won't miss 'em. You'll see.

Step 4

Carry a Bottle of Ice Water Everywhere

Staying well hydrated will help keep your blood sugar levels stable and temper cravings. Plus, you'll lose weight automatically!

Step 5

Commit to Moving More Every Day

Make movement self-motivating by doing physical activities that put a smile on your face. Then do them every day for at least 30 minutes. And the exercise doesn't have to be done all at once. Tally up 30 over the course of the day. Moving makes your muscles more sensitive to insulin so the hormone can clear glucose out of the blood and into muscle cells. Physical activity also reduces the dangerous abdominal fat that surrounds the organs, which is a top risk factor for diabetes.

Step 6

Go to Sleep Earlier

If you stay up late and wake up tired, you could be confusing the hormones that regulate appetite, triggering the release of the stress hormone cortisol and making it harder to lose weight. A wealth of research illustrates the health benefits of adequate sleep, including reducing risk of obesity and diabetes. You'll learn how to get to bed earlier and enjoy a restful night's sleep as we detail all of these steps later in this book.

14-Day No Sugar Diet Power Steps in Detail

Step 1

Determine Your Goal Weight

Calculate the number of pounds to lose to cut your diabetes risk nearly 60 percent. Studies suggest that a drop in weight of as little as 7 percent can do it. Here's how: Weigh yourself and multiply your body weight by .07 (7 percent weight loss).

EXAMPLE:
Your current weight is 200 pounds.

200
x .07
= **14 POUNDS TO LOSE**

---

200 current weight
- 14 pounds to lose
= **186 POUNDS, YOUR GOAL WEIGHT**

If you want something bad enough, you're going to get it. But you have to know exactly what you want. Now you do. Weigh yourself once a week, same day, same time for measurable feedback. Don't get discouraged by the scale. Stay committed to your weight loss goal. With every pound you lose toward your 7 percent goal you improve your chances of avoiding diabetes. Have faith in the plan and your ability. You'll get there.

Step 2

Eat Breakfast, Eat When You're Hungry, Eat Simply

Step 2 is the most powerful no-B.S. formula for losing weight and preventing diabetes. Practice these principles for the next 14 days and you'll be well on your way to mastering healthy eating habits for life. Let's break it down so you can see how it works.

Eat Breakfast

You've heard this advice before, but it really is effective and efficient for weight loss. Here's evidence:

✳ Researchers from Saint Louis University found that people who ate eggs for breakfast consumed 330 fewer calories throughout the day than those who ate a bagel. Eggs are one of the few foods that are a complete protein, containing all nine essential amino acids that your body can't make itself. Protein releases the hormone leptin that suppresses appetite.

✳ Scientists reporting in the *American Journal of Epidemiology* found that people who skipped breakfast were 4.5 times more likely to be obese than those who didn't miss the morning meal. Why? People who postpone eating until late morning or lunchtime often satisfy their ravenous hunger with sugars and processed carbohydrates. Try to get in the habit of having a breakfast that features protein (like eggs) and fiber (whole fruit and whole-wheat toast) and you'll avoid the blood-sugar dip that leads you to pastries and pizza.

✱ Another study at the University of Missouri compared the blood sugar impact of a high-protein breakfast to that of a high-carbohydrate breakfast in people with type 2 diabetes. For seven days, the participants ate either a 500-calorie high-protein breakfast meal consisting of 35 percent protein and 45 percent carbohydrate, or a 500-calorie high-carbohydrate breakfast meal consisting of 15 percent protein and 65 percent carbohydrate. On the seventh day, the breakfast meal was followed by a standard 500-calorie lunch 4 hours later, and blood samples were taken throughout the day to assess the subjects' levels of glucose, insulin, and several gut hormones that help regulate the insulin response. The researchers found that the high-protein breakfast lowered blood glucose levels after both breakfast and lunch and that insulin levels were slightly elevated after lunch, indicating that the participants' bodies were working properly to manage blood sugar.

So, you see, protein in the morning is key. But you don't have to eat a steak's worth of protein to get the blood-sugar benefits of the morning meal. Researchers say eating just 25 to 30 grams of protein at breakfast will satisfy your hunger and help keep blood sugar manageable. You can get that much protein by scrambling two large eggs and two large egg whites, drinking a banana avocado smoothie, or eating a Greek yogurt breakfast bowl made with quinoa. See chapters 8 and 9 for some breakfast suggestions.

Fiber is critical in the morning, too. Oatmeal makes a great anti-diabetes breakfast despite being high in carbs. That's because it contains lots of fiber.

Oatmeal illustrates how fiber from any vegetable, fruit, or grain works in your gut. Consider what happens when you pour hot water on your steel-cut oats: The oats soak up the water like a sponge, increasing in volume. That's what happens to fiber in your belly. It puffs up like a balloon, which slows down digestion and minimizes the impact on your blood sugar. It also keeps you feeling full longer. Now, sprinkle some slivered almonds on top of your oatmeal, suggests David Katz, MD, president of the American College of Lifestyle Medicine. "The nuts contain protein, fiber, and healthy fats that can help stabilize insulin levels."

Eat When You're Hungry

Many people don't like to eat in the early morning or they don't have time to make a proper breakfast in the rush to get to work. That's okay. Eat when you're hungry, not because the clock says it's time to eat. Just make sure you don't wait too long to eat in the morning and become so ravenous you make poor food choices or overeat.

Try this: Wait until after you get to work, say at 10 a.m., to put something high in protein and fiber in your belly. That strategy may even help you lose more weight because you are essentially reducing your "eating window" for the day, according to scientists at the Salk Institute for Biological Studies. Your "eating window" is, essentially, your waking hours. So, if you have breakfast at 7 a.m. and have your last snack at, say, 10 p.m., that's a 15-hour eating window, more opportunity to consume more calories. If you limit your eating window to between, say, 10 a.m. and 7 p.m., and skip an evening snack, you've significantly slashed your opportunities to eat by almost a third. As long as you avoid most processed carbohydrates during that window and eat belly-satisfying foods containing protein, healthy fats, and fiber, you won't be likely to overeat.

Belly-off bonus: By pushing off breakfast for a few hours, you are extending your nighttime fast. If you exercise first thing in the morning, your body will be inclined to tap fat for fuel instead of carbs because your blood sugar will automatically be lower.

Eat Simply

Simplifying your diet makes it easier to control calories and lose weight. Eating simply means not overcomplicating mealtime with too many choices. It means sticking to a routine of foods that you know are healthy for you and you know you love to eat. It's actually a very good weight-loss strategy, especially when you are making a significant change in your normal eating habits like cutting out added sugars. Find a low-sugar cereal you like and stick to it. Discover the healthiest sandwich on a fast-food menu and order that every time you go. Pick a healthy dinner you love to eat and make enough to have two nights' worth of leftovers. Too much variety can lead you down the path of overconsumption. Think about the last time you ate at a buffet. Did you fill your plate with a little taste of everything? Studies show that the more variety of foods people are offered, the more likely they are to consume more. For example, Cornell University researchers discovered that people will eat more M&M'S candies from a bowl when there is an abundant variety of colors of candies in the dish instead of just a few different colors. And a study at the University of Texas Health Science Center in 2015 found that people who ate a more diverse diet tended to have larger waist circumferences than people whose diets were less diverse.

Steps for Eating Simply

A little planning makes eating healthier and losing weight a lot easier.

■ **Purge your home of temptations.** Do a clean sweep of your fridge and pantry to get rid of the huge variety of sweets and processed foods within that will tempt you. By eliminating fast-burning processed carbs like sodas, candy, juices, baked goods, packaged products, processed snacks, and non-whole-grain white bread and pasta from your home, you'll find ways to satisfy your hunger with healthier options.

■ **Choose a handful** of the No Sugar Diet Superfoods in chapter 6 to build your weekly meals around. For the next 14 days, at least, simplify your menu to include a handful of recipes that you love that will ensure good blood sugar control and hunger satisfaction. Remember to focus on quality carbohydrates such as fresh vegetables and fruits, legumes, and whole grains, in that order. Be sure that every meal and snack contains some protein, such as fish, poultry, eggs, legumes, nuts, seeds and cheese, and red meat, in that order. Also, have a little healthy fat with each meal to boost satiety. Good sources are olive oil, avocado, nuts, fish, and cheese.

■ **Do some meal prep on Sunday evenings.** Make and freeze a batch of bean chili for quick heat-and-eat dinners. Boil a dozen eggs for hard-boiled egg snacks to take to work. Plan to pack your lunches instead of eating out. Keep in mind that the average fast-food meal weighs in at more than 600 calories. In one study published in the *Journal of the Academy of Nutrition and Dietetics*, women who brought their lunches to work lost five more pounds than dieters who went out for lunch at least once per week.

■ **Simplify your kitchen counter.** Keeping a clean, uncluttered kitchen leads to a healthier diet (and probably fewer ants). According to a study in the journal *Environment and Behavior*, people who have cluttered, messy kitchen counters strewn with chip bags, cookie boxes, and even cereal boxes tended to consume 40 percent more calories than people with tidy kitchens.

■ **Use the half-plate rule.** Practice this every time you sit down to lunch or dinner: Fill one half or more of your plate with vegetables. Fill the space that's left with mostly lean protein and the rest with whole grains or legumes. It's the easiest way to reduce calories and lose weight without counting calories, say dieticians. Because vegetables are low-calorie, high-water-content, nutrient-dense foods, they satisfy your hunger for less overall calories.

Step 3
Banish Those Sneaky Sugar Sources

Added sugars are everywhere. If you don't normally read the nutrition facts and ingredients lists of the packaged foods you buy, you won't know just how much sugar is sneaking into your diet. You can significantly slash calories and reduce the blood sugar spikes and dips that trigger cravings by becoming more mindful of the content of the foods you eat. That takes becoming a bit of a nutrition detective. Start sleuthing. Read food labels. Be aware of the hidden sugars in common foods. (The next chapter is a good place to start your education.) Do your best to avoid foods with the highest amounts of added sugars. Eventually, your taste buds will recognize when a food is just too sweet.

Step 4
Carry a Bottle of Ice Water Everywhere

Cutting out sugary beverages is the easiest, quickest way to start losing weight and lowering high blood sugar. It is so easy to swallow hundreds of calories and much too much added sugar from soft drinks over the course of a day without even noticing. Consider: A large McDonald's Sweet Tea contains 71 grams of added sugar, delivering 280 calories. An 18.5-ounce bottle of Gold Peak Sweet Tea packs 48 grams of sugar for 190 calories.

In both cases, that's a lot of sugar. So be mindful of this weight-gain pitfall and avoid it. But think about this: If you eliminated just one sweet tea or soda every day for a year, you'd cut out the calorie equivalent of nearly 20 pounds of fat. Work your way toward drinking only water or unsweetened tea. One way to do that is by swapping high-calorie, high-sugar beverages for less sweet options. The second and more preferable solution is to make your own iced tea, gradually using less and less sugar until you don't miss the sweet stuff at all. Water and unsweetened iced tea will become your go-to beverages. What's more, your desire for other sugary foods will wane, too, until cereals, condiments, and baked goods high in added sugars will be too sweet for your palate.

Drinking lots of water during the day can also make it easier to lose weight. For one, thirst is often misunderstood for hunger. Try answering a hunger pang with a zero-calorie glass of water and see how you feel five minutes later. The amount of water you drink may also impact your blood sugar levels. Not long ago, a study of 3,615 men and women conducted by the French National Research Institute found that people who drink very little water, a few glasses each day, may be more likely to develop abnormally high blood sugar. While monitoring 700 of these study participants over nine years, the researchers found that people who drank 17 ounces of water or more per day were 28 percent less likely to develop high blood sugar than those who drank less. While the study doesn't prove a cause-and-effect relationship, scientists suggest that people who drink little water may be overloading on sugary drinks, which could lead to weight gain and high blood sugar. There could be another factor at play: *vasopressin.* This hormone acts as an antidiuretic to help regulate water retention in the body. When you become dehydrated, vasopressin is produced to signal the kidneys to conserve water, which may elevate blood sugar.

Are you dehydrated? Here are some clues:

- Check your urine. Is it dark in color? You're dehydrated. Your pee should be the color of lemonade, light in color, when you are drinking enough water.

- Pinch the skin between your thumb and index finger and then let go. If you are well-hydrated, it should snap right back smooth. If the pinch lingers there, you can probably use a drink.

To drink more water each day, keep a tumbler full of ice water with you at your desk at work and take it wherever you go. Sip constantly. And remember that you get a lot of water from the foods you eat, especially fresh vegetables and fruits like lettuce, watermelon, apples, broccoli, spinach and pears.

Step 5
Commit to Moving More Every Day

Let's be honest with ourselves: We just don't move our bodies much compared to our ancestors in the days before golf carts, BarcaLoungers, Amazon Prime, and Netflix. How much of your day is spent sitting? It's pretty easy to figure out: Check in with yourself every hour for one day and write down your butt-in-chair time. Add it up. Surprised?

Researchers say the average person spends more than half of their waking hours sedentary, watching TV, sitting in a car, or working at a computer. You've probably heard about the study that made big news back in 2015 about our national sitting habit. An analysis of previous research in the *Annals of Internal Medicine* found that sitting for 8 or 9 hours a day is a health hazard. The study found that sitting for prolonged periods raises your risk for diabetes by, get this, 91 percent! How is that so? Well, jump back to what we learned in chapter 3: Physical activity helps move the sugar that's in your blood into your cells. When you sit, the sugar just stays there and increases your insulin resistance.

So, this is critical: Move more, every day. Make movement self-motivating by doing something that puts a smile on your face, like walking or tennis, or swimming. Then do it every day for at least 30 minutes. Remember that breakthrough 2002 study that outlined how to reduce the risk of diabetes nearly 60 percent? Part of the formula was logging 150 minutes of physical activity every week.

Now, maybe you are not a fan of formal exercise. A lot of people don't like it. You may think it's boring or too hard. Some people feel intimidated by going to a gym, a spin class, or a yoga studio. And that's fine. While I strongly believe you have a lot to gain by stepping out of your comfort zone and trying some new way to get moving, I realize that working out in a gym isn't for everyone. Being active and having fun doing it, however, is for everyone.

If you don't like running or lifting weights, don't do them. Find something you enjoy doing that gets you off the couch and away from the TV. Find something that's enjoyable to you that moves your legs and arms and gets your heart and lungs working harder. If you're moving, it counts toward that 30 minutes a day of physical activity that'll help you prevent diabetes.

Here are some of the endless move-more possibilities:

- Bicycling
- Roller skating
- Lap swimming
- Nature walking
- Golfing
- Zumba
- Swing, jazz, salsa, ballroom dancing
- Tai Chi
- Bowling
- Softball
- Basketball
- Gardening
- Indoor rock climbing
- Cross-country skiing
- Badminton
- Yard work
- Rowing
- Yoga
- Pilates
- Barre fitness
- Backpacking

- Fencing
- Martial arts
- Cardio kickboxing
- Spinning classes
- Rope jumping
- Fitness trampoline jumping

The secret to sticking with any fitness-boosting activity is choosing an activity that matches your personality type. Do you like group activities or do you prefer to do things by yourself? Are you competitive or collaborative? It really doesn't matter what you choose to do to get moving. This is what does matter:

• It gives you a sense of accomplishment and satisfaction.

• It elevates your heart rate and challenges your muscles—your upper and lower body.

• You can do it at a vigorous level for 30 minutes every day. Tip: You don't have to do 30 minutes all at once. Exercise experts say you can accumulate 30 minutes a day by breaking it up into, say, three 10-minute segments. Just make sure you huff and puff a bit and break a sweat.

• It's fun. If it's not enjoyable, you'll quickly find an excuse to avoid it.

Most people enjoy walking outside. So, until you find your "exercise" passion, I want you to follow the 14-Day No Sugar Diet High-Intensity Interval Training walking workout in chapter 10. As you lose weight and feel stronger, advance to the simple body-weight strength-building workout in that chapter as well. Toning your muscles will improve insulin's ability to clear glucose from your blood, reducing your risk of type 2 diabetes.

Step 6
Go to Sleep Earlier

Try this tonight: Go to bed at least 30 minutes before you normally do. Then, evaluate how you feel in the morning. I'll bet you'll feel better rested, more energetic, and happier when you wake up. Good quality sleep, and an adequate amount of it, plays a huge role in good health and stress reduction. And studies show that poor sleep habits—getting too much or too little—impact your blood sugar levels and your waistline.

Japanese researchers looked at the sleep habits of 4,870 people and monitored their body fat percentage and HbA1c test scores. They found that people who slept between 6.5 and 7.4 hours per night (which is considered a healthy duration for most people) had the lowest A1c scores, while people who slept either less than 4.5 hours or more than 8.5 hours per night had higher A1c levels regardless of physical activity or diet. In addition, people who slept for short or long durations tended to have the highest body fat.

Poor sleep throws key hormones that regulate appetite, cravings, and emotional stress levels out of whack. Tossing a monkey wrench into a smoothly running system causes a mix of problems that can lead to weight gain, inflammation, and insulin resistance. Studies show that when you are exhausted from lack of sleep, your body begins to crave sugar and fat. (Have you experienced this?) Your metabolism slows down while levels of the stress hormone corti-sol increase. In one study, women who slept less than six hours a night or more than nine hours were more likely to gain about 11 pounds compared with women who slept 7 to 8 hours a night.

Steps for Better Sleep

Good sleep is a habit you can quickly develop with a little effort and a lot of consistency.

■ **Go to bed at the same time every night.** And wake up at the same time, too. Get into a healthy routine. Start by hitting the sack 15 to 30 minutes earlier until you can consistently sleep six and a half to seven and a half hours. You should quickly feel the difference.

■ **Don't watch TV in bed.** Don't do work in bed either. Sit at a table with your laptop. Your bed should be used for only two things, sleep and sex.

■ **Tune in before you turn in.** Studies suggest that you may enjoy more satisfying sleep if you listen to music before you retire. Of course, you'll want to choose Mozart, Diana Krall, or Norah Jones instead of Metallica. Listen to music in the 60 to 80 beats-per-minute range to mimic your resting heartbeat, say researchers.

■ **Make your room pitch black.** Light entering your eyes suppresses the production of melatonin, a hormone that makes your body sleepy. Block out light from windows with room-darkening curtains, remove night lights, and turn off your smartphone. Even light from your electronic devices can disrupt sleep.

■ **Turn the temperature down.** Cooling your body induces sleep. So shed the heavy down comforter and use cotton sheets.

■ **Avoid heavy snacks before bedtime.** Have a little something like half a banana, a protein shake, or a small bowl of cereal with milk an hour and a half to two hours before bed. Walnuts work. They contain melatonin. Warm milk? Grandma was right. Milk has calcium and tryptophan, both of which your brain needs to produce melatonin. Also, the warm liquid warms your body. As your body cools, you become sleepy.

Now that you know the steps that will, over the next 14 days, put you on the right track toward preventing or reversing type 2 diabetes, let's turn to a chapter that identifies certain foods you should do your best to avoid, the most energy-dense, high-sugar foods you'll encounter each day. Eliminate or reduce these 30 foods most of the time and you will make great strides toward losing weight and maintaining healthy blood sugar levels.

Avoid or Limit These High-Sugar, High-Carb Foods

Half the battle is just being mindful of what you put in your mouth

A GARDEN SALAD with dressing. Grilled chicken. Baked beans. And a Glaceau Vitaminwater. Sound fairly healthy to you? That was my dinner at an end-of-summer cookout at my friend Eric's place on Labor Day. I felt pretty good about my choices, especially when I said no thank you to the hamburger bun for my chicken, the potato chips, and the bottle of craft beer he offered. I was watching my carbs.

Then, after drenching my salad with the fat-free sun-dried tomato vinaigrette, I glanced at the nutrition label on the bottle. Huh, 12 grams of sugar—more than I expected. The ingredients list explained why: high fructose corn syrup. Then I checked my pink Vitaminwater bottle. Whoa! 32 grams of sugar. That's 8 teaspoons. At home, I looked up the sugar content of those baked beans: 12 grams. Add in the two generous squeezes of barbecue sauce I squirted onto my chicken breast, and I figured my meal would have hit 68 grams of sugar, as sweet as eating 30 Willy Wonka Pixy Stix candies. Luckily, I swapped my Vitaminwater for a Coors Light and saved 20 grams.

It doesn't take a degree in nutrition science to figure out that your frosted pink jelly doughnut with multi-colored sprinkles is loaded with sugar. But it's very easy to allow the sugars in many other foods to go unnoticed—and sneak into your bloodstream.

As you've learned in this book, certain foods that contain a lot of sugar and carbohydrates and make your blood sugar spike rapidly can act as an appetite stimulant. When your body releases insulin to help push the influx of sugar that's in your blood into your cells, sometimes your blood sugar drops too low, too quickly, and you feel weak and hungry for more sugar. That's a sugar cycle to avoid, and you can, by being mindful of the sugars in the foods you eat and eliminating those foods from your diet or at least minimizing them.

A quick glance at where you'll find high amounts of carbohydrates and sugars in common foods:

	Serving size	Carbs	Sugars
Ketchup	1 Tbsp	4.5 g	3.7 g
Wheat crackers	6 crackers	20 g	1 g
Jelly doughnut	1 doughnut	32 g	14 g
Plain bagel	1 bagel	46 g	9 g
Fast-food cheeseburger	1 small	33 g	7 g
Jarred pasta sauce	½ cup	13 g	10 g
Granola bar	1 bar	18 g	8 g
Banana	1 large	31 g	17 g
Corn muffin	1 large	58 g	8 g
Microwaveable tomato soup	1 cup	20 g	14 g
Orange juice (fresh squeezed)	1 cup	27 g	21 g
Peach yogurt	1 container	32 g	25 g

(Number of grams will vary by brand.)

Maybe some of those foods surprise you. That's my point: Sugars are everywhere. If you want to get off the roller coaster of blood sugar spikes that cause cravings and start losing weight quickly, it really helps to be a sugar sleuth and be disciplined about avoiding the most notorious culprits. Work toward becoming a more mindful eater. Think before you swallow. Do some investigative work when you go food shopping by reading nutrition labels and targeting calories, carbs, and sugars. (See Name Your Poison on page

56.) And get to know some of these common foods that pack the lion's share of carbohydrates and added sugars—some containing 20 grams or more.

Applesauce

Remember that no one ever said "an applesauce a day keeps the doctor away." You're better off eating an apple than going for the pureed version. One cup of sweetened applesauce contains 36 grams of sugar but only 3 grams of fiber. A medium-size apple, on the other hand, has 4 grams of fiber and, although still sweet, only has 19 grams of sugar. And apples are rich in cancer-fighting antioxidants.

Banana

Bananas are a good source of magnesium, a nutrient that aids protein synthesis, which, in turn, increases lean muscle mass. Magnesium also helps boost lipolysis, the process by which the body releases fat from its stores. And, of course, it's one of the best sources of potassium, which lowers blood pressure. Bananas, therefore, are good for you. But they are high in carbs at 31 grams per large fruit. So have a banana, but not a whole bunch. In fact, half a banana may be enough to satisfy you.

Barbecue Sauce

Condiments can be tricky, and measuring out portion size isn't always an option. The next time you order ribs off the menu, keep in mind that just two tablespoons of barbecue sauce can contain upward of 11 grams of sugar. In a restaurant, you can expect that more than four tablespoons are slathered onto a serving of ribs.

Candy

Many people think of fruity, fat-free candies like Twizzlers, Sour Patch Kids, and gummy bears as better-for-you candies, but the truth is they're just as packed with carbs and sugar as their chocolate counterparts—and in some cases, they actually carry more carbs. For example, a pack of M&M'S Brand Candy carries 34 grams of carbs, while a packet of Sour Patch Kids is packed with 52 grams. And just four Twizzlers Twists (which the brand considers a standard serving size) contain 36 grams of carbohydrates. If you're looking for a lower-carb sweet, consider grabbing a handful of Life Savers Gummies. Eight of them have 22 grams of carbs. But you'd be better off with a few grapes or raspberries. Try them frozen.

Canned Fruit Cocktail

Fresh fruit has natural sugars from fructose, so they are most beneficial when you need an extra energy burst. However, there's no good time to eat canned fruits, which are often packed in high fructose corn syrup. A one-cup serving of canned peaches, for example, can contain upward of 39 grams of sugar. If you need your fruit to last longer, head to the freezer aisle and reach for no-sugar-added varieties that were flash-frozen at the peak of their ripeness.

Canned Soup

You probably know to be wary of sodium in canned soup, but you may not know that many varieties are riddled with sugar, too. Campbell's Slow Kettle Style Tomato & Sweet Basil Bisque, for example, has 24 grams of sugar per cup. Sure, some of that is coming from the tomatoes, but that's still a lot of sweetness in which to dunk your grilled cheese.

Chocolate Milk

While its high carbohydrate and protein content often inspires personal trainers to call chocolate milk the perfect recovery drink, it's still high in sugar. "Dairy contributes naturally occurring lactose, but many brands add sweeteners along with the chocolate flavor," says Cara Harbstreet, MS, RD, of Street Smart Nutrition. "Unless you're highly active or engaging in intense exercise, those added calories might not provide many benefits." For daily sipping, reach for a glass of plain low-fat or whole milk and pair it with a small piece of dark chocolate to satisfy your sweet tooth.

Cranberry Sauce

Come Thanksgiving Day, let's all promise to do without this wobbly, gelatinous, too-sweet sauce. A half-cup serving contains 56 grams of carbohydrates and 48 grams of sugars. Turkey Day wouldn't be the same, you say? Then take a tablespoon only and call it a day.

Energy Bars

Since carbs provide energy, it should come as no surprise that energy bars are loaded with carbohydrates. Still, a lot of people think these health-food imposters are actually good for you. Not so. On average, they contain up to 45 grams of carbohydrates—and are chock-full of sugar and scary chemicals, too. They're basically a triple threat to your health.

Energy Drinks

Most of these so-called performance drinks are loaded with sugar and caffeine. Example: One can of Red Bull contains 27 grams of sugar. That's more than you'd find in six Dunkin' Donuts sugar-raised doughnuts.

Flavored Kefir

Drinking kefir is a good way to boost good-for-you gut bacteria. But stick to the unflavored kind. The fruity flavors are very, very sweet. Some contain up to 22 grams of sugar per serving. Unsweetened kefir contains fewer than half of those sugar grams. Here's an idea: Buy both kinds and mix a little of the flavored kefir with the unflavored to reduce the sugar content of your beverage.

Flavored Teas

Sweet tea and other high-sugar flavored teas in a bottle are not better for you than soda just because they have "tea" in their names. Many of them contain nearly 46 grams of sugar per bottle!

Flavored Iced Coffees

These can pass as liquid candy, too. A bottle of Starbucks Frappuccino contains 37 grams of carbs and 31 grams of sugar, delivering 200 calories per serving.

French Fries

While most people know that potatoes are starchy, French fries are extremely carb-laden at 63 grams per restaurant serving, twice as many carbs as a bowl of pasta in a standard family-style serving. It gets worse: Vegetable-oil-fried foods like fries contain high levels of something called inflammatory advanced glycation end products (AGEs), which are inflammation-causing compounds that form when certain foods are cooked at high temperatures.

Fresh-Pressed Juices

Organic, fresh-pressed juices might sound innocent, but don't depend on them for health benefits. Guzzle down just one glass, and you'll be drinking a sugar bomb with as many as 26 grams. And though you are getting the juice of whole fruit, you're not getting the fiber of the whole fruit. Without the fiber from the plant, the juice isn't much better than drinking a cup of sugar water.

"Healthy" Frozen Dinners

When you're in a pinch, reaching for a frozen meal might not sound like a bad option—especially when that meal is labeled "healthy." Still, pay attention to nutrition labels. Healthy Choice's Café Steamers Pineapple Chicken, for example, touts grilled white meat and protein-rich edamame among its ingredients but has a whopping 19 grams of sugar in one bowl—more than the 18 grams of protein it contains.

Low-Fat Yogurt

Low-fat yogurts are exceptionally high in sugar. Brands use it in excess to distract you from the lack of fat. You might expect fruit-filled yogurt to be high in sugar—like Strawberry flavored Yoplait and Dannon's Fruit-on-the-Bottom Blueberry, which contain 26 grams and 24 grams, respectively—but "healthy" yogurts are, too. Surprisingly Stonyfield Organic Smooth & Creamy Low Fat Vanilla contains

29 grams of sugar, and All Natural Non-Fat Brown Cow Vanilla has 25 grams. Activia Blueberry Probiotic is not far behind at 19 grams. Yoplait Thick and Creamy Key Lime Yogurt contains 28 grams of sugar, as much as 4 Chips Ahoy! Chewy cookies. Opt for plain Greek yogurt and add your own berries.

Maple Syrup

You know that maple syrup is packed with sugar, but who'd have thought that going organic could be even worse than the gross, fake kind. (We're looking at you, Mrs. Butterworth!) Madhava Organic Maple Agave Pancake Syrup delivers 30 grams of sugar in just two tablespoons. The only upside? The flavor of organic syrups is stronger and more concentrated than the high-fructose-made syrups, so you don't need to use as much.

Margarita Frozen Cocktail

While whipping up a frozen margarita at home isn't quite as bad as getting it from a bar (400 calories vs. 700), it's still the worst possible cocktail for your waistline. Made with a sugar-spiked neon mix and tequila, the summer staple will overload your system with more sugar than you'd find in nine Dunkin' Donuts Apple n' Spice Donuts! Other frozen beverages aren't much better. The average strawberry daiquiri, for example, has about 280 calories and 44 grams of sugar per serving. Not to mention, it's also 99 percent high fructose corn syrup. Switch to a glass of sparkling wine with muddled strawberries and lemon slices to get your fruity fix for a fraction of the waist-widening sugar grams and calories.

Muffins

Just one commercially prepared blueberry muffin has as many carbs as not one, not two, but five slices of bread! It's also a fat and calorie mine, carrying over 520 calories and a third of the day's fat in one pastry. And eating half now and "saving the rest for later" is nearly impossible; foods rich in carbs, fat, and sugar are downright addicting. A University of Montreal study found that mice who had been fed diets with high levels of those very nutrients displayed withdrawal symptoms and were more sensitive to stressful situations after they were put on a healthier diet. Don't think you can fix the problem by ordering a "bran muffin." The minimal fiber inside is no match for the sugar crush. One Dunkin' Donuts Honey Bran Muffin contains 39 grams of sugar per serving, on par with a doughnut.

Pie

You knew this holiday-time staple was indulgent, but thanks to all the added sugar and fruit-filled centers, a slice of the dessert manages to serve up more carbs than a bowl of pasta.

Pizza

If you can't live without pizza, well, you're not trying very hard. But, really, if you enjoy pizza, at least top your slice with lots of vegetables to boost the fiber profile. At 36 grams of carbohydrate, each slice is like eating a bowl of penne pasta.

Quinoa

Packed with the hunger-busting combo of 8 grams of protein and 6 grams of fiber in just one cooked cup, quinoa is good stuff. Just keep an eye on your portion sizes. A cup contains nearly 40 grams of carbohydrates. Instead of thinking of quinoa as the "main attraction" on your plate, consider it more as a topping. Sprinkle it on top of salads, add it to your omelets, or use it in lieu of a sugar-filled granola in Greek yogurt parfaits.

Raisins

This sweet and chewy oatmeal topper carries 34 grams of carbs—just slightly more than a cup of penne—in one tiny single-serve box. Unlike dried fruit, fresh fruit contains water, so grapes make for a far more filling snack.

Fat-Free Salad Dressing

Products that boast the claims "low-fat" or "fat-free" are usually code for "high in sugar." When manufacturers take the fat out of food, they make up for the lost flavor with extra salt and sugar, usually about 12 grams of the latter per serving. The fats in salad dressings like Newman's Own are usually the heart-healthy monounsaturated fats found in olive oils, and there's no need to take these out. Try Newman's Own Balsamic Vinaigrette. It tastes sweet but only contains 3 grams of carbs and 1 gram of sugar per 2-tablespoon serving.

White Bread

Packaged white bread can have 4 grams of sugar per slice. That means you'd be eating 8 grams of sugar per sandwich—

more sugar than a pack of jelly beans. To make things worse, it is often sweetened with high fructose corn syrup, one of the most flat-belly-threatening forms of sugar on the market. If you typically go with wraps because you think they're healthier than bread, you've got things all wrong. Wraps can have about the same number of carbs as two slices of white bread. What's more, to keep the big tortilla flexible, manufacturers often add soybean oil and hydrogenated oils. Go with Ezekiel's sugar-free, sprouted grain loaf. The millet, spelt, lentils, and cholesterol-lowering barley lend a natural sweetness and help boost the loaf's fiber, a nutrient that wards off hunger while keeping the nutrient profile sound. Plus, sprouting grains break down enzyme inhibitors, which helps your body better digest and absorb healthy nutrients from the bread.

Smoothies

Bottled fruit smoothies seem healthful, but if you do a little nutrition facts investigation, you'll see that they are almost as calorie, carb, and sugar heavy as a milkshake. The no-sugar-added bottled varieties by Naked, for example, pack anywhere from 44 to 55 grams of carbs per bottle. Make your own smoothies with protein powder. Check out the recipes in chapter 8.

Soy Milk

Although cow's milk contains natural sugar from lactose, the sugar in non-dairy milk is often the added kind. And at 19 grams per cup, chocolate soy milk really pushes the sugar boundary. Choose unsweetened or light varieties.

Soda

You already knew 12 ounces of soda was filled with chemicals and about 10 teaspoons of sugar, but did you realize that it packs more carbohydrates than an entire bowl of pasta? It's true. A 12-ounce can of Sprite has 38 grams of carbs, while a classic cola has about 39 grams.

Whole-Wheat Pancakes

When it comes to eating a stack of pancakes, you might know you're getting ready for carb overload, but sugar doesn't always register. After all, if you skip the butter and fruit compote, you should be fine, right? Not always. A stack of four Harvest Grain 'N Nut Pancakes from IHOP might sound healthier than buttermilk, but they actually contain 26 grams of sugar. Add on some light maple syrup, and you're looking at 30-plus grams in your morning meal.

Name Your Poison
How to spot hidden sweeteners on an ingredients list

You say muscovado, I say turbinado. No matter how you pro-
nounce it, our bodies know it's sugar. You might not recognize
some of the types of sugar that food manufacturers use to sweeten processed foods. Keep an eye out for these lurking on ingredients lists:

- Agave nectar
- Barley malt
- Beet sugar
- Brown sugar
- Cane juice
- Caramel
- Carob syrup
- Corn syrup
- Dextrose
- Fructose
- Fruit juice concentrate
- High fructose corn syrup (HFCS)
- Honey
- Malt syrup
- Maltodextrin
- Maltose
- Molasses
- Muscovado
- Rice syrup
- Saccharose
- Sucrose
- Turbinado sugar

Steer Away from Breakfast Cereals

Avoid a bowl of added sugars; find a better morning meal

Sure, they are easy to fix in the morning rush, but most are little more than sugar in a box despite the claims of being "part of a nutritious breakfast." While you might expect to find a lot of carbs in General Mills Cocoa Puffs (you're right, 23 g carbohydrates and 9 g sugars), you might be surprised to learn that the healthier-sounding Kellogg's Smart Start Strong Heart Original Antioxidants has nearly triple (65 g carbohydrates, 21 g sugars). The ingredients lists tells the story: rice, wheat, oat clusters, sugar, high fructose corn syrup, molasses, honey, polydextrose, and corn syrup. Healthy-sounding cereals can make your blood sugar soar. So, read labels. Better yet, cut cereals out of your diet. There are better foods for breakfast.

A Cereal Sampler

- **Kellogg's Raisin Bran** (9 g sugars)

- **General Mills Reese's Puffs** (13.5 g sugars)

- **Instant Cream of Wheat, Apples 'n' Cinnamon** (16 g sugars)

- **General Mills Golden Grahams** (13.5 g sugars)

- **Quaker Oatmeal Squares** (13 g sugars)

- **Kashi Strawberry Fields** (11 g sugars)

- **Post Honeycomb** (7 g sugars)

- **Quaker Natural Granola Oats & Honey** (26 g sugars)

- **Kellogg's Cracklin' Oat Bran** (19 g sugars)

- **Quaker Instant Oatmeal, Cinnamon Roll** (13 g sugars)

CHAPTER

6

Superfoods for a Bulletproof Body

Keep your kitchen filled with these powerful foods that help regulate blood sugar, stop cravings, and burn fat

OUT OF SIGHT, out of belly. If you want to stop snacking on your kids' pretzel sticks, keep them off the kitchen counter. If you want to beat your doughnut addiction into submission, don't allow these sugar bombs in the house. Make "out of sight, out of belly" your mantra whenever you restock your kitchen with food for the week. If cookies and chips no longer exist in your home, you can't eat them—that is, unless you make a special trip to the store. And who's going to do that? Research shows that if blood-sugar-spiking foods are not within reach in your pantry, in your fridge, or on your kitchen counter, you're less likely to eat them. The flip side is also true: If foods that fight cravings, keep blood sugar stable, and help you lose weight are at hand, you'll eat the good stuff.

So, stock up on the delicious foods that will help you in your effort to slash added sugars and beat diabetes. Use the superfoods in this chapter to make up your shopping list. Then create tasty breakfasts, lunches, dinners, and snacks with them.

Know Your Macros

Our calories come from three macronutrients: carbohydrates, proteins, and fats.

Carbohydrates are energy-boosting foods like fresh vegetables and fruits, legumes, and whole grains. These are good quality carbohydrates because they are not processed or just minimally processed and contain an important blood-sugar-regulating ingredient: dietary fiber. You don't have to count carbohydrate grams (most people find that too cumbersome), just try to eat most of your calories from whole, fiber-rich carbohydrates. Tip: Make vegetables, especially colorful ones and leafy greens, half to three-quarters of your plate.

We also get our carbohydrates from highly processed foods like cereals, baked goods, soda, and other sweetened beverages, white bread, white rice, and non-whole-grain pasta—the low-fiber foods you found in the previous chapter. Limit these blood-sugar-raising foods as much as you can. Try to avoid them completely.

Proteins. Fish, poultry, eggs, legumes, nuts, seeds, cheese, and red meat are all good proteins. Make them fill up about a quarter of your meal plate. Some proteins also contain some fat, so keep that in mind as you fill your plate. Tip: Having some protein at every meal and snack will help satisfy your hunger longer to clobber cravings.

Fats. These are not the bad guys we once thought they were. In fact, even saturated fats are acceptable in moderation because they are so satisfying, helping us to reduce overall calories by keeping us fuller longer. Olive oil, avocado, nuts, and fish are examples of monounsaturated fats (often called MUFAs) that are heart healthy.

On the following pages are examples of the best high-quality, fiber-rich, energy-boosting carbohydrates, satiating proteins and healthy fats. For recipes that incorporate these superfoods, see chapter 9.

Eat Simple Tip

■ Some people find that eating the same basic recipes each week makes meal planning and weight loss easier, especially during the initial weeks of a switch to healthier eating. Select a handful of your favorite superfoods and recipes and plan out your meals for the week. By keeping things simple, you'll be more likely to stick to your plan and avoid meals that break the rules of the 14-Day No Sugar Diet.

✳ Vegetables and Fruits

It's the simplest weight-loss and beat diabetes rule: Make vegetables fill most of your plate. Whole fresh vegetables are all good low-calorie sources of vitamins, minerals, and fiber. But some starchy vegetables like potatoes, corn, and butternut squash contain more carbs than non-starchy vegetables like leafy greens, broccoli, radishes, sugar snap peas, and Brussels sprouts do. Fill up on the non-starchy variety and practice portion control with the more starchy veggies.

Artichoke Hearts

The easiest way to get this antioxidant-rich vegetable in your diet is by using canned or jarred artichoke hearts, because the fresh variety takes forever to prepare. (Just be sure to rinse off the artichokes if they have been swimming in a bath of added sodium.) With 14.4 grams of fiber per cup, cooked, for a mere 89 calories, this vegetable makes a light yet tasty, filling addition to salads and chickpea or lentil pasta.

Broccoli

Broccoli is one of the best vegetables you can eat because it is a terrific source of vitamin C, fiber, folate, and phytochemicals that have been associated with reduced rates of cancers in the lung, colon, and bladder. Like cauliflower and Brussels sprouts, it's a cruciferous vegetable containing a powerful anti-cancer compound called sulforaphane. Now, research suggests it may help reverse the progression of type 2 diabetes. In a recent Swedish test-tube study done on liver cells of diabetic rats, sulforaphane reduced the glucose production of those liver cells. In another study, this time on humans, broccoli sprout extract given to obese patients with type 2 diabetes significantly reduced their fasting blood glucose and HbA1c scores versus control subjects.

Brussels Sprouts

Like broccoli, these mini cabbages are rich in sulforaphane as well as antioxidants that can help detoxify cancer-causing free radicals, and 80 percent of your daily vitamin C in just ½ cup.

Butternut Squash

Don't avoid this starchy vegetable just because it's sweet and high in carbs. The blood-sugar rush you might expect is lessened by the amount of fiber it contains: almost 7 grams per cup of baked squash. Besides flavor and fiber, you're getting very high amounts of the powerful antioxidants vitamins A, C, and E. Also, roasted acorn squash contains 3 grams of fiber per serving.

Celery

Here's another high-water-content, low-calorie food that's great in salads and soups, or simply eaten raw. Studies suggest that it might be a powerful anti-diabetes vegetable due to the vitamin K inside. Vitamin K, a strong anti-inflammatory, may improve your sensitivity to insulin, helping you metabolize blood sugar. In a 2010 study in *Diabetes Care*, researchers looked at the diets of more than 38,000 people and found that those with the highest consumption of vitamin K–rich foods had a lower risk of type 2 diabetes than people who consumed the least vitamin K.

Leafy Greens

One of the best ways to control your blood sugar is to follow the diabetes plate method, which calls for filling half your plate with non-starchy veggies, a quarter with a grain or starchy veggie, and a quarter with a lean protein. "This method helps keep calories in check, portions satisfying, and nutrients high," says nutritionist Jackie Newgent, RD. "Greens like kale and spinach are great non-starchy vegetable options because they contain lutein, an important nutrient for eye health. This nutrient is essential for people with diabetes since they have a higher risk for blindness than those without diabetes." Other ideal leafy greens include Swiss chard, romaine lettuce, and Boston or Bibb lettuce.

Peppers

Peppers have a high water content, so they fill you up for little calorie or carb impact. Red, orange, and green peppers are anti-inflammatory superfoods—but go red to reap the most benefits. Out of the three colors of bell pepper, red has the highest amount of inflammatory-biomarker-reducing vitamin C along with the bioflavonoids beta-carotene, quercetin, and luteolin, according to research in the *Journal of Food Science*. Luteolin has been found to neutralize free radicals and reduce inflammation. Beta-carotene is a carotenoid, a fat-soluble compound that is associated with a reduction in a wide range of cancers, as well as reduced risk and severity of inflammatory conditions, such as asthma and rheumatoid arthritis.

Spinach

Spinach is extremely low in both calories and carbohydrates, with just 7 calories and 5 grams of carbs per cup, so it makes an excellent weight-loss food. In fact, it's so low in both that you can almost call it a "free food" that you can eat as much of as you'd like without increasing your diabetes risk. Spinach is also a rich source of plant-based omega-3 fats and folate, extremely important nutrients; both help reduce the risk of heart disease, stroke, and osteoporosis. Spinach is also packed with lutein, a compound that fights age-related macular degeneration.

Fruit

Eat whole fresh fruits, not those pureed into high-calorie smoothies either in your home blender or a manufacturer's bottle. Also, avoid dried fruits most of the time due to their high sugar content.

Apples

People who ate at least two servings each week of certain whole fruits—particularly apples, blueberries, and grapes—reduced their risk for type 2 diabetes by as much as 23 percent in comparison to those who ate less, according to research in the *British Medical Journal*. Apples are a good source of dietary fiber and phytochemicals that have strong antioxidant and anticancer properties.

Blueberries and Other Berries

A study in the *Journal of Nutrition* found that when people who were at risk for type 2 diabetes took ingredients found in blueberries daily, their sensitivity to insulin improved, which reduced their risk of developing diabetes. Blueberries and other berries (strawberries, blackberries, and raspberries) are all low on the glycemic index (GI), meaning they have less impact on your blood sugar.

Pears

Just one medium fruit with the skin on is enough to fulfill a quarter of your daily needs of fiber. This fall fruit also helps to keep hunger at bay thanks to a soluble fiber called pectin that attracts water and turns to gel, slowing down digestion, which may help to reduce blood sugar and cholesterol.

Cherries

Cherries contain naturally occurring chemicals called anthocyanins that could reduce insulin production by 50 percent, according to a study in the *Journal of Agricultural and Food Chemistry*.

Watermelon

Watermelon is a good example of a food that has a high glycemic index (GI) but is actually fine for people with high blood sugar. High-GI foods typically cause a faster rise in blood glucose. But because watermelon is high in water and fiber, the sweet fruit actually has not much effect on blood sugar levels. It has a low glycemic load (GL), which is another rating system that's a better measure of expected blood glucose response because it factors in the amount of carbohydrates. A half-cup serving of watermelon contains just 5 grams of carbohydrates. Just be careful about portion sizes; it's easy to overeat this sweet, juicy fruit.

✳ Proteins

When choosing proteins, it's important to pay attention to their carbohydrate and fat content. While grilled and baked meats are typically low in carbs, plant-based proteins (like beans), as well as breaded and fried meats, contain carbs. With that in mind, it's best to read food labels carefully before digging into these foods so you can portion your servings properly.

"Char-grilled, burnt meats damage cell membranes and insulin receptors that are associated with insulin resistance," cautions nutritionist Miriam Jacobson, MS, RD. A little bit of char is inevitable when you're grilling, but if any parts are extremely blackened, cut them off before eating, suggests the American Diabetes Association.

Beans and Lentils

Dried beans and lentils provide a solid combination of plant protein and soluble fiber that can help boost feelings of fullness and help manage blood sugar levels. Replacing some meat with beans or lentils can play a helpful role in heart health, which is of particular importance for people with diabetes. Not sure how to include them in your diet? Try garbanzo beans, kidney beans, black beans, mung beans, and lentils in salads, soups, casseroles, and chili. Or puree them into hummus.

Chickpeas and Hummus

Along with other legumes, chickpeas are high in fiber and protein, which helps them increase feelings of fullness. A number of studies have shown that people on a reduced-calorie diet who eat chickpeas in salads and soups or hummus spread lose more weight and have lower cholesterol than people who don't eat chickpeas. Legumes make you feel fuller longer by causing your body to release an appetite-suppressing hormone called cholecystokinin.

Eggs

Many studies have shown that people who eat protein for breakfast, specifically eggs, consume fewer calories afterwards for up to 36 hours. That's proof of the satiating power of protein. Eating eggs reduces the insulin response after the meal. And it works. A study published in 2008 in the *International Journal of Obesity* found overweight and obese people given two eggs a day for breakfast lost 65 percent more weight than those eating a similar breakfast without eggs.

Greek Yogurt

Avoid most flavored yogurts, many of which have less than 7 grams of protein and are loaded with added sugars. Plain Greek yogurt is a proven weight-loss winner: Vitamin D and calcium unite to shut down the belly-flab-producing hormone cortisol, while the high protein content helps build fat-torching lean muscle mass. As long as you skip over the fat-free variety (2% will keep you feeling fuller) and stick with plain (fruit or honey = dessert), you've got a rich-tasting snack with a reasonable amount of sugar. I like plain Fage Total 2% yogurt; it has only 8 grams of sugars. I mix in slivered almonds and shelled sunflower seeds for crunch and blueberries for flavor.

Cool Your Hunger with Water

■ **Are you drinking enough water?** Research has shown that people often mistake hunger for thirst. Next time you feel a pang of hunger, down a glass of ice water and wait a few minutes. Your cravings for food will likely go away.

Plant-Based Protein or Whey Protein Powders

Protein is critical for maintaining healthy body composition, blood sugar balance, and muscle growth. But eating it at every meal and snack, as prescribed in the No Sugar Diet, can be challenging. Enter protein powders, which make it easier to build more protein into your day. Plant-based protein and whey protein powders mix easily in water, almond milk or yogurt for quick, belly-satisfying snacks. A University of Toronto study found that eating whey protein before a meal provided satiety signals that prevented a group of healthy young adults from overeating.

Meats

Meats such as poultry, beef, pork, veal, and lamb contain no carbohydrates, so they do not raise blood glucose levels. Try to choose the leanest portions available and keep serving size to between 2 and 5 ounces. For chicken and turkey, remove the skin before eating to reduce the saturated fats and cholesterol. Limit the amount of red meat you eat. Recent research from the Harvard School of Public Health suggests a regular diet of red meat increases your risk of type 2 diabetes. Harvard researchers looked at three large studies of male and female healthcare professionals who were followed for between 14 and 28 years. They found that a daily serving of red meat boosted risk of developing type 2 diabetes by 19 percent. What's worse, processed red meats like hot dogs and bacon eaten daily were associated with a 51 percent increased risk. "We don't need to remove red meat from the diet entirely," says Harvard researcher Frank Hu, PhD. "Americans just need to move meat from the center of the plate to the side of the plate."

Wild Salmon

"Salmon is a smart addition to anyone's eating plan, but for individuals with diabetes, it's especially beneficial," says Lori Zanini, RD, of Lori Zanini Nutrition in Los Angeles. Here's why: "It's a healthy protein source that will not raise blood sugar levels and will help to lower 'bad' choles-

---

HELPFUL TECHNIQUES

Control Your Portions

It's important to be mindful of the amount of carbohydrates, sugars, and calories in a food when you are trying to manage your blood sugar and lose weight. That doesn't mean you have to count them. Here are some tips to use as guidelines.

Eyeball method: When choosing a packaged food, such as a box of cereal, read the nutrition label and make sure the food has at least 3 grams of fiber and fewer than 10 grams of sugar.

Portion estimation: For women—1 palm-size portion of protein-dense food per meal; 1 fist-size portion of vegetables (or more vegetables if you are having no grains, potatoes, or legumes); 1 cupped hand of carb-dense foods like grains or potatoes; 1 thumb-size portion of fat. For men—2 palms' worth of dense protein; 2 fists' worth of vegetables; 2 cupped hands of carb-dense foods, like grains or potatoes; 2 thumbs' worth of fats.

---

terol levels, which increases the risk of heart disease and stroke—a major concern for diabetics."

✳ Whole Grains

According to the American Diabetes Association, it's impor tant to choose the most nutritious whole grains possible. Although grains help to maintain steady blood-sugar levels and provide fiber, white flour–based products can't claim the same. Because the bran, germ, and endosperm have been compromised, these foods elevate blood-sugar levels and should only be consumed on occasion.

Oats

"Oats contain a type of fiber called beta-glucan, which seems to have an anti-diabetic effect," explains Jackie Newgent, RDN, CDN, author of *The All-Natural Diabetes Cookbook*. "I advise people with diabetes to steer clear of added sugars by enjoying savory rather than sweet oatmeal."

Quinoa

This nutty, trendy whole grain is a good source of fiber and protein, making a smart pick for a diabetes prevention diet. "With the fiber and protein combination found in quinoa, you'll feel fuller and have better blood sugar control," says dietician Sarah Koszyk, RDN. "The protein in quinoa also helps with the uptake of carbohydrates so the body can process them more easily. I suggest enjoying quinoa in a salad or casserole." Just be careful of portion size because, as a grain, it naturally contains a lot of carbs.

Whole-Grain or Ezekiel Bread and Whole-Grain Pasta

You can have bread, but just not the white kind, says Lori Zanini, RD. "White sandwich bread is a refined grain, not a whole grain. When eaten as is, it has a high glycemic index and can directly lead to elevated blood-sugar levels." Swap out white bread for whole-grain or Ezekiel bread and choose whole-grain pasta or a legume-based pasta made from chickpeas or lentils in lieu of regular nutrient-stripped noodles.

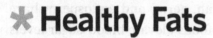 Healthy Fats

Avocado

This creamy, delicious fruit contains a significant amount of healthful monounsaturated fats and dietary fiber, which help slow the release of sugars into the bloodstream, prompting less insulin to be needed. Avocados also contain a unique weight-loss-friendly carbohydrate called mannoheptulose that research links to lower insulin secretions and a compound called beta-sitosterol that quells inflammation.

Olive Oil

Rich in the same monounsaturated fat found in avocados, olive oil fights insulin resistance and encourages the release of the appetite-suppressing hormone leptin.

Nuts, Nut Butters, and Seeds

Researchers from the Harvard School of Public Health discovered that women who consumed nuts or peanut butter five times a week or more lowered their risk for type 2 diabetes by nearly 30 percent compared to those who rarely or never ate nuts or peanut butter. But all peanut butters and other nut butters are not created equal. Many contain added sugars. And roasted nuts are high in substances called advanced glycation end products that damage cell receptors and encourage insulin resistance. Raw nuts are a much better choice.

Almonds, Raw

A good source of protein, healthy fats, and fiber, raw almonds don't raise blood sugar and they are particularly high in magnesium, a nutrient that improves insulin sensitivity.

Chia Seeds

This ancient grain plumps up in your stomach, making you feel fuller and slowing digestion to temper rises in blood sugar levels after meals. The tiny seeds are anti-inflammatory agents that contain omega-3 fats, magnesium, folate, iron, and potassium, all useful against metabolic syndrome.

Ground Flaxseed

Sprinkle this on oatmeal, salads, soups, or in smoothies. Ground flaxseeds contain lignans (a plant-based chemical compound) and fiber, which help maintain blood sugar levels. Flaxseed is also rich in thiamine, magnesium, copper, phosphorus, and manganese.

Nut Butters

Peanut butter has the highest protein content of the nut

butters, but it is often mixed with hydrogenated oil, added sugars and preservatives, so read labels carefully and opt for natural peanut butter when you can find it.

Almond butter contains more heart-healthy mono-unsaturated fats than the other nut butters. Read labels and choose almond butter that lists "almonds" as the sole ingredient.

Cashew butter is typically higher in sugar and lower in protein than either peanut or almond butter. Make it better by pureeing raw, unsalted cashews in a food processor.

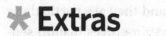 Extras

Here are some other useful items that can help you manage your glucose levels and weight:

Cinnamon

Boost the flavor of your food and help lower blood sugar. Sprinkle cinnamon on your yogurt and hot cereal. Add some to ground coffee before brewing. A 2003 study in the journal *Diabetes Care* showed that cinnamon might cause muscle and liver cells to respond more efficiently to insulin. This improves blood sugar balance and helps with weight loss. Research has shown that Ceylon cinnamon, in particular, seems to reduce several risk factors for cardio-vascular disease, including high blood sugar and levels of triglycerides, LDL ("bad") cholesterol, and total choles-terol. Studies suggest that just ½ teaspoon a day for 20 days is enough to improve your insulin response and lower blood sugar by up to 20 percent.

Green Tea

This zero-calorie beverage has been shown to prevent over-eating, stabilize blood sugar levels, rev up our metabolism, and reduce fat storage. In a Penn State University study, obese mice that were fed EGCG, a compound found in green tea, along with a high-fat diet gained weight more slowly than mice that did not receive the green tea supplement.

Vinegar

Be sure to add vinegar to your sandwiches. Put it in salad dressing or sprinkle it on steamed vegetables or even meats. Research in the *European Journal of Clinical Nutrition* has shown that vinegar taken before or after a high-carbohydrate meal reduces blood sugar spikes and increases in insulin and creates a sense of fullness. In another study, researchers at Arizona State University found that people who started a meal with a vinegar drink enjoyed better blood sugar and insulin profiles following meals. The high acetic acid content in vinegar deactivates an enzyme called amylase that turns starch into sugar. Vinegar also boosts the body's sensitivity to insulin, improving blood sugar control. The best vinegars for managing glucose levels are white or apple cider vinegar. Balsamic vinegars aren't the best because they contain more sugar.

Coffee

If you drink it black (no sugar or creamer), coffee is a fine drink for people looking to prevent diabetes. Some studies suggest caffeinated or decaf brew may reduce your risk of type 2 diabetes, according to the Mayo Clinic. But watch the sugar. A single sugar packet contains 4 grams of carbs and most people use much more than one packet. If you are already diabetic, your doctor may advise you to avoid coffee because caffeine's effect on insulin function may impact blood sugar.

Turmeric

This orange-yellow spice is a powerful anti-inflammatory with diabetes-fighting properties. Other spices like fenugreek seed, cumin, ginger, mustard, onion, and coriander also seem to be anti-diabetic.

Sugar Fact

According to the *Journal of the American Dietetic Association,* the top three sources of added sweeteners in the typical American diet are:

- Soft drinks (33%)
- Solid sugars, such as table sugar, syrups, candies, jams, and jellies (16%)
- Baked goods, such as cookies, pastries, and cakes (13%)

CHAPTER

7

The 14-Day No Sugar Diet Meal Plan

What to eat for the next two weeks to lose weight and feel great

WHEN STARTING a healthy eating program, some people like suggestions for exactly what to eat when. If that's you, this 14-day meal plan on the following pages will start you off on the right track. Or use it as a general guide and pull in other recommended recipes from chapter 9 that appeal to you.

Some helpful notes before following this plan:

On Counting Calories.

- Counting calories, and grams of carbohydrates, protein, fat, and fiber, is kind of unpleasant. It sort of turns mealtime into math homework for me, so I don't do it. What's more, studies have demonstrated that nutrition information on most food labels is inaccurate and may be off by as much as 25 percent. That's another reason why I don't normally add up the numbers when I eat. However, I do eyeball these nutrition numbers on occasion. Even if they aren't perfectly accurate, I find that the nutrition facts help me to be aware of the general makeup of a meal so I can be more mindful of my food choices and portion sizes. I wouldn't recommend calorie counting; it's a hassle. But I do encourage everyone to practice mindful eating and that means understanding what's in your food.

- A more useful tool, I find, is the hand method of guesstimating how much of each macronutrient to eat at a given meal. You may find it "handier" than calorie counting, too. (See Helpful Techniques: Control Your Portions on page 70.)

On Total Calories.

- You'll find daily calorie totals below each menu list. Without an evening snack (which is optional), each day delivers roughly 1,500 calories. You will lose weight on that moderately low-calorie diet.

- Men, depending on their size, may require a few hundred more calories per day. You can easily adjust by taking a slightly larger portion size, or adding a little more protein and fat and more vegetables, whole grains or fruit, or an evening snack.

- Man or woman, if you still feel hungry after a meal, have a second glass of water and wait five or 10 minutes. Usually hunger will subside. If still hungry, have some more vegetables to fill up. The goal is to learn to listen to your body's hunger cues and make adjustments according to your body's needs. Strengthening your mindful eating skills is the secret to long-term weight-loss (and blood sugar control) success.

On Being Prepared.

- It's easier to eat healthy when you have healthy food to eat. At the start of your 14-Day No Sugar Diet, go food shopping to stock up on the ingredients you'll need to prepare healthy meals.

- Tip: Start the plan on a Monday. The day before, prepare some snacks and meals for the week. Doing so will help you avoid rushing out for fast food when hunger strikes and healthy alternatives aren't at hand.

On Being Realistic.

- Dining out is an enjoyable experience. There's no reason to sacrifice that part of your life. Just be realistic. Restaurants serve oversize portions of calorie-dense foods. You can still go out to eat on occasion and follow the No Sugar Diet if you simply recognize that being handed a menu is not a pass to stop eating mindfully. Go with a plan. Know what you want to order before you arrive and keep portion size and meal content in mind. And remember to ...

- begin your meal with a tall glass of water
- send back the breadbasket
- start with an appetizer of broth-based soup or salad
- don't rush through the meal
- be sure your plate includes protein, a little fat, and mostly vegetables.

14-Day
Sample Meal Plan

DAY 1

BREAKFAST
Spinach & Cheese Omelet (recipe page 119)
1 slice whole-wheat toast with butter

SNACK
Handful of walnuts or raw almonds
190 calories, 18 g fat (2 g sat.), 4 g carbohydrates, 4 g protein, 2 g fiber

LUNCH
Greek Salad (recipe page 126)

SNACK
Hummus & Pepper Roll-Ups

YOU'LL NEED:

2   Tbsp. hummus
1   8-inch low-carb, multi-grain tortilla
½   red bell pepper, sliced

DO THIS:

• Spread hummus on tortilla.
• Top with slices of red bell pepper, roll up and cut into wheels.

170 calories, 6.8 g fat (3 g sat.), 22 g carbohydrates,
6.5 g protein, 5.8 g fiber

DINNER
Chicken Parmesan (recipe page 134)
Add 2 oz. lentil and quinoa spaghetti with ½ cup marinara sauce
Add garden salad or steamed broccoli

SNACK (optional)

BEVERAGES

Eight or more eight-ounce glasses of water per day.

_ _ _ _ _ _ _ _ + water

(Other beverages: unsweetened coffee, tea, or iced tea, fruit and herb-infused waters)

Day 1 Nutrition Total (approx.)

1,469 calories, 68 g fat (19.6 g saturated),
184 g carbohydrates, 93 g protein, 27 g fiber

DAY 2

BREAKFAST
Oatmeal & Berries (recipe page 119)

SNACK
Key Lime Pie Smoothie (recipe page 109)

LUNCH
Roast Beef and Horseradish Wrap (recipe page 128)
Homemade potato salad with egg and mayonnaise

SNACK
5 baby carrots with 2 Tbsp. chickpea hummus

DINNER
Chicken & Vegetable Kebabs with Quinoa (recipe page 136)
1 slice watermelon

SNACK (optional)

BEVERAGES

Eight or more eight-ounce glasses of water per day.

__ __ __ __ __ __ __ __ + water

(Other beverages: unsweetened coffee, tea, or iced tea, fruit and herb infused waters)

Day 2 **Nutrition Total** (approx.)

1,450 calories, 44 g fat (6.4 g saturated), 98 g carbohydrates, 101 g protein, 26.8 g fiber

---

DAY 3

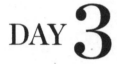

BREAKFAST

Fiber One Original Cereal with ½ cup skim milk and fresh blueberries
186 calories, 1.2 g fat, 52 g carbohydrates, 7.2 g protein, 17 g fiber

SNACK

Small pear and low-fat cheese stick
146 calories, 4 g fat (2 g sat.), 23 g carbohydrates, 6.5 g protein, 5 g fiber

LUNCH

Turkey Avocado Sandwich (recipe below) with
Cream of Tomato Soup (recipe page 126)

YOU'LL NEED:

2 tsp. spicy brown mustard
2 slices sprouted grain bread
4 slices roasted turkey breast
3 slices avocado
   Arugula leaves

Makes 1 serving.

307 calories, 15 g fat (1.8 g sat.), 21 g carbohydrates, 18.6 g protein, 5.5 g fiber

SNACK
1 cup popcorn and ½ cup skim milk
74 calories, .62 g fat, 12 g carbohydrates, 5.2 g protein, 1.2 g fiber

DINNER
Cod with Romesco Sauce (recipe page 136)
With brown rice and green beans
226 calories, 1.8 g fat (0.4 g sat.), 44 g carbohydrates, 5 g protein,
3.5 g fiber
Strawberries with whipped cream
204 calories, 6.6 g fat (6.6 g sat.), 34 g carbohydrates, .9 g protein,
1.1 g fiber

SNACK (optional)

BEVERAGES
Eight or more eight-ounce glasses of water per day.

_ _ _ _ _ _ _ _ + water

(Other beverages: unsweetened coffee, tea, or iced tea, fruit and herb
infused waters)

Day 3 **Nutrition Total** (approx.)
1,587 calories, 50 g fat (13 g saturated), 201 g carbohydrates,
73 g protein, 36 g fiber

DAY 4

BREAKFAST
Drink Your Oatmeal (recipe page 108)

SNACK
Fruit Salad with Lime and Mint (recipe page 122)

LUNCH
Chicken Salad Roll-Ups (recipe page 125) **with Cream of Tomato Soup**
(recipe page 126)

SNACK

Slices of ½ of red bell pepper, 3 baby carrots for dipping in ¼ cup guacamole
170 calories, 10.6 g fat (1.4 g sat.), 18.8 carbohydrates, 3.6 g protein, 9 g fiber

DINNER

Diner-Style Meatloaf (recipe page 137) **with Kale and Cannellini Beans** (recipe page 135)
Strawberries with whipped cream
204 calories, 6.6 g fat (6.6 g sat.), 34 g carbohydrates, .9 g protein, 1.1 g fiber

SNACK (optional)

BEVERAGES

Eight or more eight-ounce glasses of water per day.

_ _ _ _ _ _ _ _ + water

(Other beverages: unsweetened coffee, tea, or iced tea, fruit and herb infused waters)

Day 4 **Nutrition Total** (approx.)

1,614 calories, 61 g fat (15 g saturated), 201 g carbohydrates, 65.5 g protein, 29.1 g fiber

---

DAY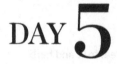

BREAKFAST

Breakfast Burrito (recipe page 115)

SNACK

1 medium banana with Tbsp. of almond butter
206 calories, 9.5 g fat (.9 g sat.), 30.4 g carbohydrates, 3.4 g protein, 3.6 g fiber

LUNCH

Chick-Fil-A Grilled Chicken Cool Wrap

350 calories, 14 g fat (5 g sat.), 29 g carbohydrates, 3 g sugars,
37 g protein, 15 g fiber

SNACK

Mini Muffin Pizza

YOU'LL NEED:

1   whole-grain English muffin
2   slices tomato
4   Tbsp. shredded mozzarella cheese
    Red pepper flakes (optional)

DO THIS:

- Top two halves of a whole-grain English muffin with a slice of tomato
  and shredded mozzarella cheese.
- Place in a toaster oven or under a broiler and heat until the cheese is
  melted. Sprinkle with red pepper flakes.

280 calories, 6 g fat (3 g sat.), 44 g carbohydrates, 15 g protein, 8 g fiber

DINNER

Planked Salmon with Grilled Asparagus and Roasted New Potatoes
(recipe page 140)

SNACK (optional)

BEVERAGES

Eight or more eight-ounce glasses of water per day.

_ _ _ _ _ _ _ _ + water

(Other beverages: unsweetened coffee, tea, or iced tea, fruit and herb
infused waters)

Day 5 Nutrition Total (approx.)

1,623 calories, 61.5 g fat (15.4 g saturated), 175 g carbohydrates,
133 g protein, 33.6 g fiber

DAY 6

BREAKFAST
Fiber One Original Cereal with ½ cup skim milk and fresh blueberries
186 calories, 1.2 g fat, 52 g carbohydrates, 7.2 g protein, 17 g fiber
Medium Apple with 1 Tbsp. Almond Butter
143 calories, 9.5 g fat (.5 g sat.), 17.4 g carbohydrates, 2.4 g protein,
3 g fiber

SNACK
Small pear and low-fat cheese stick
Per serving: 146 calories, 4 g fat (2 g sat.), 23 g carbohydrates,
6.5 g protein, 5 g fiber

LUNCH
Chicken Salad Roll-Ups (recipe page 125)
Chipotle Sweet Potato Soup

YOU'LL NEED:

1   cup baked sweet potato (mashed)
½   cup vegetable broth
½   cup unsweetened almond milk
½   tsp. chipotle powder
      Salt to taste
⅓   cup diced avocado

DO THIS:

- Place the potato with the broth and almond milk in a blender. Blend on low until smooth.
- Add the chipotle powder and salt to taste.
- Garnish with diced avocado.

Makes 1 serving.

259 calories, 3 g fat, 47 g carbohydrates, 12 g protein, 7 g fiber

SNACK

Tuna salad tea sandwiches: Top two rye crisp crackers each with a
heaping tablespoon of light homemade tuna salad and top each with a
½-inch-thick slice of cucumber.
98 calories, 3 g fat (1 g sat.), 9 g carbohydrates, 6 g protein, 3 g fiber

DINNER

Chicken Gumbo (recipe page 133) **with 1 slice Ezekiel Sprouted Grain
bread and garden salad**
294 calories, 12.5 g fat (2 g sat.), 28 g carbohydrates, 17 g protein,
6 g fiber
Half a banana dipped in 1 oz. melted dark chocolate
77 calories, 10 g fat, 30 g carbohydrates, 2 g protein, 3 g fiber

SNACK (optional)

BEVERAGES

Eight or more eight-ounce glasses of water per day.

_ _ _ _ _ _ _ _ + water

(Other beverages: unsweetened coffee, tea, or iced tea, fruit and herb
infused waters)

Day 6 **Nutrition Total** (approx.)

1,578 calories, 40 g fat (6.5 g saturated), 204 g carbohydrates,
83.5 g protein, 17 g fiber

DAY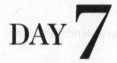

BREAKFAST

Eggs Florentine with Sun-Dried Tomato Pesto (recipe page 116)
Fruit Salad with Lime and Mint (recipe page 122)

SNACK
Yogurt with Fruit and Almonds

YOU'LL NEED:

½ cup blackberries
½ cup raspberries
¼ cup All Bran cereal
1 Tbsp. sliced almonds
½ cup plain Greek yogurt

DO THIS:

- Mix all together.

Makes 1 serving.

231 calories, 8.5 g fat (2 g sat.), 14.7 g protein, 3 g fiber

LUNCH
Tuna Salad Wrapped in Lettuce (recipe page 144)
Melon Slush (recipe page 122)

SNACK
Half a banana dipped in 1 oz. melted dark chocolate.
77 calories, 10 g fat, 30 g carbohydrates, 2 g protein, 3 g fiber

DINNER
Salmon Burger with Dill (recipe page 142)
Black Bean Salad with Avocado (recipe page 124)

SNACK (optional)

BEVERAGES
Eight or more eight-ounce glasses of water per day.

_ _ _ _ _ _ _ + water

(Other beverages: unsweetened coffee, tea, or iced tea, fruit and herb infused waters)

Day 7 **Nutrition Total** (approx.)
1,469 calories, 40.5 g fat (10 g saturated), 126 g carbohydrates, 81.7 g protein, 25 g fiber

DAY 8

BREAKFAST
Oatmeal & Berries (recipe page 119)
1 hard-boiled egg
77 calories, 5 g fat (2 g sat.), 1 g carbohydrates, 6 g protein

SNACK
Endless Summer Smoothie (recipe page 108)
Handful of raw almonds
162 calories, 14 g fat (1 g sat.), 6 g carbohydrates, 6 g protein, 3 g fiber

LUNCH
Avocado Salad (recipe page 124)
Medium apple with 1 Tbsp. almond butter
143 calories, 9.5 g fat (.5 g sat.), 17.4 g carbohydrates,
2.4 g protein, 3 g fiber

SNACK
Strawberries with whipped cream
204 calories, 6.6 g fat (6.6 g sat.), 34 g carbohydrates, .9 g protein,
1.1 g fiber

DINNER
Portobello Turkey Burger & Bruschetta (recipe page 127)
Roasted Brussels Sprouts (recipe page 141)

SNACK (optional)

BEVERAGES
Eight or more eight-ounce glasses of water per day.

_ _ _ _ _ _ _ _ + water

(Other beverages: unsweetened coffee, tea, or iced tea, fruit and herb
infused waters)

Day 8 **Nutrition Total** (approx.)

1,443 calories, 72.9 g fat (10 g saturated), 90.5 g carbohydrates, 64 g protein, 47 g fiber

DAY 9

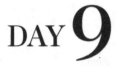

BREAKFAST
Breakfast Quinoa (recipe page 115)

SNACK
Slices of ½ red pepper, 3 baby carrots for dipping in ¼ cup guacamole
170 calories, 10.6 g fat (1.4 g sat.), 18.8 carbohydrates, 3.6 g protein, 9 g fiber

LUNCH
Leftover turkey burger and Watermelon Salad with Yogurt (recipe page 130)

SNACK
Devilishly Good Eggs (recipe page 121)

DINNER
Shrimp & Clams Stew (recipe page 143), **plus side salad and roll**

SNACK (optional)

BEVERAGES
Eight or more eight-ounce glasses of water per day.

_ _ _ _ _ _ _ _ + water

(Other beverages: unsweetened coffee, tea, or iced tea, fruit and herb infused waters)

Day 9 **Nutrition Total** (approx.)

1,458 calories, 45.6 g fat (13.4 g saturated), 126 g carbohydrates, 94 g protein, 24.5 g fiber

DAY 10

BREAKFAST
Oatmeal & Berries (recipe page 119)
1 hard-boiled egg
77 calories, 5 g fat (2 g sat.), 1 g carbohydrate, 6 g protein

SNACK
Douse the Flames Smoothie (recipe page 107)

LUNCH
Tex-Mex Bean Salad (recipe page 129)
Medium apple
80 calories, 30 g carbohydrates, 4 g fiber

SNACK
5 baby carrots with chickpea hummus
107 calories, 2.8 g fat, 17 g carbohydrates, 4.6 protein, 16 g fiber

DINNER
Flank Steak Salad (recipe page 139) **with whole-grain roll and salad**
540 calories, 17 g fat (7 g sat.), 32 g carbohydrates, 41 g protein, 6 g fiber
2 tangerines
74 calories, 16 g carbohydrates, 1.2 g protein, 2.5 g fiber

SNACK (optional)

BEVERAGES
Eight or more eight-ounce glasses of water per day.

__ __ __ __ __ __ __ __ + water

(Other beverages: unsweetened coffee, tea, or iced tea, fruit and herb infused waters)

Day 10 **Nutrition Total** (approx.)
1,476 calories, 45.8 g fat (10.5 g saturated), 169 g carbohydrates, 88.6 g protein, 44 g fiber

DAY 11

BREAKFAST
Huevos Rancheros (recipe page 117)

SNACK
Oatmeal with Berries and Almond Butter

YOU'LL NEED:

- 1 cup steel-cut oatmeal
- ½ cup fresh raspberries
- 1 Tbsp. almond butter

DO THIS:

- Cook the oatmeal and then mix in berries and almond butter.

285 calories, 20 g fat (3.5 g sat.), 34 g carbohydrates,
12.5 g protein, 11 g fiber

LUNCH
Tequila Sunrise Salad (recipe page 144)

SNACK
Hummus & Pepper Roll-Ups

YOU'LL NEED:

- 2 Tbsp. hummus
- 1 8-inch low-carb, multi-grain tortilla
- ½ red bell pepper, sliced

DO THIS:

- Spread hummus on tortilla.
- Top with slices of red bell pepper, roll up and cut into wheels.

170 calories, 6.8 g fat (3 g sat.), 22 g carbohydrates,
6.5 g protein, 5.8 g fiber

DINNER
Eggplant Parmesan (recipe page 138)
Strawberry Pecan Salad (recipe page 128)

SNACK (optional)

BEVERAGES
Eight or more eight-ounce glasses of water per day.

__ __ __ __ __ __ __ __ + water

(Other beverages: unsweetened coffee, tea, or iced tea, fruit and herb infused waters)

Day 11 Nutrition Total (approx.)
1,503 calories, 89.2 g fat (15.5 g saturated), 103.4 g carbohydrates, 65 g protein, 48.8 g fiber

---

DAY 12

BREAKFAST
Huevos Sedona (recipe page 118)

SNACK
Small pear and low-fat cheese stick
146 calories, 4 g fat (2 g sat.), 23 g carbohydrates, 6.5 g protein, 5 g fiber

LUNCH
Pesto Chicken Sandwich (recipe page 139)
Melon Slush (recipe page 122)

SNACK
Strawberry-Kiwi-Almond Crunch Yogurt

YOU'LL NEED:

½ cup Greek yogurt, plain
½ cup strawberries, sliced
2 peeled kiwifruit, chopped
3 Tbsp. sliced almonds

DO THIS:

- Mix the first three ingredients and then top with sliced almonds.

318 calories, 10 g fat, 39 g carbohydrates, 23 g protein, 8 g fiber

DINNER
White Bean Soup with Sausage (recipe page 145)

SNACK (optional)

BEVERAGES
Eight or more eight-ounce glasses of water per day.

_ _ _ _ _ _ _ _ + water

(Other beverages: unsweetened coffee, tea, or iced tea, fruit and herb infused waters)

Day 12 Nutrition Total (approx.)
1,452 calories, 67 g fat (14.5 g saturated), 196 g carbohydrates, 87 g protein, 58 g fiber

---

DAY 13

BREAKFAST
Spinach & Cheese Omelet (recipe page 119)

SNACK

Handful of walnuts or raw almonds
190 calories, 18 g fat (2 g sat.), 4 g carbohydrates, 4 g protein, 2 g fiber
Kale and Apples Smoothie (recipe page 108)

LUNCH

Tuna Salad Wrapped in Lettuce (recipe page 144)

SNACK

Small pear and low-fat cheese stick
146 calories, 4 g fat (2 g sat.), 23 g carbohydrates, 6.5 g protein, 5 g fiber

DINNER

Chicken Chili (recipe page 132) **with side salad and whole-grain roll**
Fruit Salad with Lime and Mint (recipe page 122)

SNACK (optional)

BEVERAGES

Eight or more eight-ounce glasses of water per day.

_ _ _ _ _ _ _ _ + water

(Other beverages: unsweetened coffee, tea, or iced tea, fruit and herb
infused waters)

Day 13 **Nutrition Total** (approx.)

1,360 calories, 49 g fat (13.5 g saturated), 121 g carbohydrates,
80 g protein, 23 g fiber

DAY 14

BREAKFAST

Eggs Florentine with Sun-Dried Tomato Pesto (recipe page 116), **plus**
whole-wheat toast and ½ red grapefruit

SNACK

Key Lime Pie Smoothie (recipe page 109)

LUNCH
Leftover Chicken Chili with whole-wheat roll and side salad

SNACK
Hummus & Pepper Roll-Ups

YOU'LL NEED:

2 Tbsp. hummus
1 8-inch low-carb, multi-grain tortilla
½ red bell pepper, sliced

DO THIS:

- Spread hummus on tortilla.
- Top with slices of red bell pepper, roll up and cut into wheels

210 calories, 6.8 g fat (3 g sat.), 22 g carbohydrates,
6.5 g protein, 5.8 g fiber

DINNER
Planked Salmon with Grilled Asparagus and Roasted New Potatoes
(recipe page 140)

SNACK (optional)

BEVERAGES
Eight or more eight-ounce glasses of water per day.

__ __ __ __ __ __ __ + water

(Other beverages: unsweetened coffee, tea, or iced tea, fruit and herb
infused waters)

Day 14 **Nutrition Total** (approx.)
1,459 calories, 27.8 g fat (8 g saturated), 109 g carbohydrates,
114 g protein, 21.7 g fiber

No Sugar Diet Smoothies

Quench your hunger with a quick and satisfying treat

HOW 'BOUT a smoothie? A thick, rich, delicious shake as a snack or meal replacement is another useful weapon in the war against diabetes. Before you grab a straw, however, there's something you should know: Smoothies enjoy a misleading "health halo" that could backfire on you. *Smoothie* doesn't *always* translate to *healthy*. Just because these frothy drinks may be made with virtuous stuff—whole fruit, juice, yogurt, milk, and protein powder—they could blend together into a sugar-laden calorie bomb that spikes your blood glucose as high as if you had just gorged on jelly beans.

So, don't lay down your guard at the blender in your kitchen and especially not at the fast-food counter. Adding peanut butter and chocolate syrup, for example, can double the sugar and calorie load, sending a surge of glucose into your bloodstream, definitely not good for someone with prediabetes or diabetes. Beware: Some large restaurant-made smoothies pack 700 or more calories and over 63 grams of sugar. That's more sugar than you'd get by eating 20 Ginger Snap cookies! Here's another image to plant in your mind's eye: Imagine yourself pushing a lawnmower from one end of a football field to the other on a hot summer day. You'd have to do that about 100 times to burn off the calories in some large restaurant smoothies.

Beat Diabetes Tip

◼ Eating a whole fruit is almost always better than drinking a fruit smoothie. The fiber in whole fruit acts like a braking system to slow down the process of turning fructose from the food into blood sugar.

Okay, *now* you can grab a straw. Because by drinking specific "No Sugar Diet smoothies" made right, as this chapter's recipes demonstrate, you'll enjoy one of the healthiest and tastiest ways to flatten your belly and lower your risk of diabetes. What's the trick? Adding protein, healthy fats (avocado, seeds, and nuts), and even more fiber into the blender to slow the uptake of sugars into the bloodstream during digestion.

The No Sugar Diet Smoothie Rules

1) **Avoid juice as a liquid base.** Even 100% fruit juice contains loads of sugar. Instead, use water, milk, or a milk substitute, such as almond milk. Cow's milk is relatively high in sugar, but it's a better choice than fruit juices.

2) **Don't add sugars** in the form of honey, maple syrup, or agave syrup. Gradually adjust your taste buds to enjoy unsweetened beverages and foods. If you need to sweeten your smoothie, try stevia, a natural sweetener. But use very little; stevia is 40 times sweeter than table sugar.

3) **Use low-sugar fruits** such as berries and others. (See the low-sugar fruit list on page 103.) These fruits add sweetness to your drink with minimal fructose, plus they add fiber and vitamins. Remember to go easy on fruit. Even though it contains the fiber of whole fruit, once pulverized, it absorbs more quickly. And, as you know, you can down a smoothie in a fraction of the time it takes to eat a whole piece of fruit, meaning faster uptake of sugars. If you use a fruit from the high-sugar list (page 106), use a quarter to no more than half of the fruit serving and only that one fruit.

4) **Add protein.** Unsweetened Greek yogurt and plant-, egg-, or whey-based protein powders are easy ways to boost the protein profile of your smoothie. Remember: Protein slows digestion and builds muscle. (See

suggestions for good protein powders on pages 110 and 111, which include an explanation of the benefits of each.)

5) **Add green fiber.** Experiment with adding leafy greens to your smoothies. It's a great way to get more vegetables in your diet, boost the fiber content of your shakes, and get more helpful nutrients. For example, adding spinach to your smoothie can stifle hunger and cravings, thanks to compounds in the leafy green's cells that promote the release of satiety hormones. You can also add chia seeds or hemp seed nuts. The latter contain 6 grams of high-quality protein per tablespoon. That's more than beef or fish.

Sugar Fact

■ A 15.2-ounce bottle of 100% orange juice contains 42 grams of sugar, about as many sugar grams as in 16 Bite-Size Famous Amos Chocolate Chip Cookies.

Low-Sugar Fruits
For Smoothies (Choose these)

Apple

Total Sugars: 1 cup, chopped, 13 g
Fiber: 3 g

Apples are a great smoothie fruit—and a terrific snack for people with insulin resistance—because they are high in fiber to slow the blood-sugar spike.

Avocado

Total Sugars: ⅓ medium, 0 g
Fiber: 3 g

Yes, an avocado is a fruit. It adds no sugar but 5 grams of healthy monounsaturated fat, plus about 20 vitamins and minerals.

Blackberries

Total Sugars: 1 cup, 7 g
Fiber: 7.6 g

The dark color of this particular berry tips you off to its high anti-oxidant content. These lush-looking berries help protect against heart disease and fight against age-related cognitive decline.

Blueberries

Total Sugars: 1 cup, 14.7 g
Fiber: 3.6 g

Though a bit higher in sugar than other popular fruits used in smoothies, blueberries are high in fiber and well known for phytonutrients called anthocyanins, which protect cells from oxidative stress.

Cantaloupe

Total Sugars: **1 cup, cubes, 9.4 g**
Fiber: **0.6 g**

Cantaloupe makes the list thanks to its extremely high water content. It's also a good source of blood-pressure-lowering potassium.

Cranberries

Total Sugars: **1 cup, whole, 4.3 g**
Fiber: **3.6 g**

In an analysis of the cancer-fighting phenol antioxidant content of 20 fruits, cranberries were found to have the highest amount.

Kiwifruit

Total Sugars: **1 fruit, pieces, 6.8 g**
Fiber: **2.3 g**

This fuzzy fruit is loaded with vitamin C and contains a good amount of magnesium, a nutrient that people with type 2 diabetes tend to lose. Magnesium supplementation has been shown to improve insulin sensitivity.

Peach

Total Sugars: **1 cup, slices, 12.9 g**
Fiber: **2.3 g**

This juicy stone fruit contains phenolic compounds that modulate different expressions of genes to ward off obesity, high cholesterol, inflammation, and diabetes.

Pear

Total Sugars: **1 cup, slices, 13.7 g**
Fiber: **4.3 g**

Pears help keep hunger at bay thanks to pectin, a soluble fiber that attracts water and turns to gel, slowing down digestion.

Raspberries

Total Sugars: **1 cup, 5.4 g**
Fiber: **8 g**

Think of raspberries as nature's magical weight-loss pill. They pack the highest fiber content of all the traditional low-sugar smoothie fruits to help boost feelings of satiety without doing any damage to your waistline.

Strawberries

Total Sugars: **1 cup, halves, 7.4 g**
Fiber: **3 g**

Nature's candy is loaded with vitamin C for immune-system strength, and it's high in water content and fiber, making it a great fruit for weight management.

Watermelon

Total Sugars: **1 cup, diced, 9.4 g**
Fiber: **0.6 g**

Watermelon is an excellent fruit for people watching their sugars because it has very little impact on blood sugar despite its sweet flavor.

High-Sugar Fruits Used in Smoothies (limit these)

Banana

Total Sugars: **1 cup, sliced, 18.3 g**
Fiber: **3.9 g**

Bananas are often used in smoothies because they add sweetness and a creamy texture. But they are rather high in sugar and carbs. When blending them, use half a medium banana and be sure to add protein and a healthy fat to slow down the absorption of sugar into the bloodstream.

Mango

Total Sugars: **1 cup, pieces, 22.5 g**
Fiber: **2.6 g**

Yes, it's high in sugars, but it's also rich in vitamins and the antioxidants quercetin, isoquercitrin, astragalin, fisetin, gallic acid, and methyl gallate—which protect the body against colon, breast, prostate cancer and leukemia. When using in a smoothie, make sure you add a healthy scoop of protein powder and a handful of raw oats to slow the breakdown of sugars.

Pineapple

Total Sugars: **1 cup, chunks, 16.3 g**
Fiber: **2.3 g**

This tropical fruit is rich in vitamins A and C, and manganese, a trace mineral that is essential for energy production. Try to use no more than a half cup in your smoothies due to their high sugar content.

Low-Sugar Smoothie Recipes

Almond Strawberry Swirl Smoothie

5   medium strawberries
1   cup unsweetened almond milk
½   cup low-fat plain Greek yogurt
5   ice cubes

• Combine ingredients in a blender and blend on high until smooth.
  Garnish glass with a strawberry slice.

No need for protein powder here. The Greek yogurt supplies enough.

Makes 1 serving.

167 calories, 6 g fat (1 g saturated), 11 g carbohydrates, 6 g sugars,
16 g protein, 2 g fiber

Douse the Flames Smoothie

1   cup unsweetened almond milk
¾   cup frozen berries (your choice)
     Large handful of fresh/frozen spinach or kale
1   Tbsp. chia seeds
1   serving vanilla plant-based protein powder
     Dash of turmeric
     Dash of cinnamon

• Combine ingredients in a blender and blend on high until smooth.

The turmeric and greens turn this into a powerful anti-inflammatory
smoothie.

Makes 1 serving.

249 calories, 8 g fat (1 g saturated), 21 g carbohydrates, 8 g sugars,
25 g protein, 7 g fiber

Drink Your Oatmeal Smoothie

½ cup blueberries
½ cup unsweetened oatmeal, cooked
½ cup Greek yogurt
1 tsp. chia seeds
Water as needed to thin consistency

• Combine all ingredients and blend, adding water to achieve desired consistency.

Makes 1 serving.

271 calories, 4 g fat (.5 g saturated), 44 g carbohydrates,
12 g sugars, 18 g protein, 7 g fiber

Endless Summer Smoothie

¼ cup 1 % milk
¾ cup seedless watermelon cubes
½ cup strawberries
½ cup low-fat Greek yogurt
2 tsp. vanilla protein powder
3 ice cubes

Makes 1 serving.

110 calories, 1.5 g fat (0.5 g saturated), 18 g carbohydrates, 10 g sugars,
8 g protein, 1 g fiber

Kale and Apples Smoothie

1 cup Granny Smith apple, quartered and seeded
½ cup frozen pineapple chunks
4 kale leaves
¼ cup fresh parley
1 Tbsp. fresh lemon juice
½ cup coconut water
½ cup water
1 cup ice

• Puree all the ingredients in a blender. Divide between two glasses.

This antioxidant-rich drink is sweet and refreshing, thanks to the sugar content of the pineapple. If you'd like to cut out some of the sugar, experiment with reducing the amount of fruit slightly.

Makes 2 servings.

Per serving: 70 calories, 0 g fat, 18 g carbohydrates, 13 g sugars, 2 g protein, 3 g fiber

Key Lime Pie Smoothie

½   cup fat-free cottage cheese
1   scoop vanilla plant-based protein powder
1   Tbsp. Key lime juice (or regular lime juice)
5   ice cubes
½   cup water
     Handful of spinach
1   Tbsp. sugar-free vanilla instant pudding mix
1   graham cracker, crushed

• Combine all ingredients except graham cracker crumbs in blender and blend until creamy. Pour into a glass. Top with graham cracker crumbs.

Makes 1 serving.

180 calories, 0 g fat, 7 g carbohydrates, 4 g sugars, 36 g protein, 0.5 g fiber

Royal Blueberry Smoothie

6   fresh basil leaves
1   cup frozen blueberries
1¾   cups almond milk
4–5 ice cubes

• Blend everything on high until smooth. Garnish with an extra basil leaf.

Makes 2 servings.

Per serving: 70 calories, 3 g fat (0 g saturated), 10 g carbohydrates, 6 g sugars, 1 g protein, 3 g fiber

Protein Powder Power

Get to know the types of protein powders and how they can help you get more of this macronutrient into your diet

Adding protein powder to a smoothie slows down the impact of the drink's carbs on your blood sugar. It also provides the building blocks of muscle repair and growth. Choosing a protein powder supplement can be a little daunting when you face the many options in a health food store or supermarket. This quick guide will help you pick the right protein for you.

There are two main types of protein supplements:

- **Animal-based protein made from whey, casein, or eggs**

- **Plant-based forms from pea, hemp, rice, and soy proteins**

Both are solid choices. Studies show that vegetable proteins may have a more powerful weight-loss effect than animal proteins. And because they're lactose-free and usually lower in sugar, vegan proteins do a better job of fighting bloat and inflammation. Milk proteins, such as whey and casein, have the ability to preserve lean muscle mass and improve metabolic health during weight loss, according to the journal *Nutrition & Metabolism*.

Any good protein powder will provide at least 15 grams of protein per serving. Here are some popular brands to consider:

Plant-Based Proteins

Sunwarrior Warrior Blend Raw Protein Powder, Chocolate

Protein source: Pea, hemp, cranberry protein, brown rice, and more
Protein payoff: 19 grams per serving

This clean protein is loaded with six servings of greens, probiotics, antioxidants, and 50 percent of your daily intake of food-based vitamins and minerals.

Garden of Life Raw Protein

Protein source: Organic sprouted protein blend (brown rice, amaranth, quinoa, millet, and more)
Protein payoff: 34 grams per serving

This complete protein powder contains 13 raw, organic sprouts, plus tea and cinnamon extract. Add a healthy fat like nut butter or avocado to your smoothie so you can absorb the fat-soluble vitamins A, D, E, and K.

Animal-Based Proteins

Promix Grass-Fed Whey Protein

Protein source: Grass-fed whey protein concentrate
Protein payoff: 25 grams per serving

Whey protein concentrate contains bioactive compounds found in the milk fat that boost metabolism and immunity.

Naked Casein

Protein source: Casein from U.S. dairy farms
Protein payoff: 26 grams per serving

Casein, as opposed to whey, digests more slowly and stays in the system longer to nourish muscles.

Paleo Protein Pure Egg

Protein source: GMO-free egg whites
Protein payoff: 25.2 grams per serving

Egg-white protein is naturally low-carb and non-fat.

CHAPTER
9

The No Sugar Diet Recipes

More than 40 ways to eat what you love while consuming less sugar

WHY DO we love recipes so? Because they are like being given permission to use a cheat sheet on a chemistry exam. You don't have to remember all the nitty-gritty details if you have the formulas right in front of you. Just follow along and you'll be rewarded with the desired result: an A+.

Consider this chapter a cheat sheet that is going to help you reach your goal weight and ace the 14-Day No Sugar Diet. Inside, you'll find more than 40 delicious breakfasts, lunches, snacks, and dinner recipes to use in your 14-Day program. By cooking more meals at home instead of eating at restaurants, you'll gain greater control over the calories and added sugars you're consuming, and you'll significantly improve the nutritional value of your meals. No thinking involved. Just make these comforting, filling, delicious recipes that have been preselected for their low sugar, high protein, and high fiber content. Enjoy!

Breakfasts

Breakfast Burrito

1   egg plus 4 egg whites, beaten
⅓   cup fresh cilantro, chopped
½   cup Canadian bacon, diced
1   whole-wheat tortilla
¼   cup shredded low-fat cheddar cheese
2   Tbsp. salsa

- Coat a skillet with cooking spray.
- Whisk the eggs together with the chopped cilantro.
- Sauté the diced Canadian bacon over medium-high heat until it begins to brown. Remove the ham to a clean bowl.
- Cook the eggs.
- Spoon the bacon into the tortilla, and then add the eggs. Top with the cheese and salsa, and fold over.

Makes 1 serving.

Per serving: 346 calories, 10 g fat (4 g saturated), 26 g carbohydrates, 3 g sugars, 43 g protein, 2 g fiber

Breakfast Quinoa

1   cup unsweetened almond milk
1   cup water
1   cup quinoa, rinsed
1   Tbsp. butter
1   cup blueberries
1   cup strawberries, sliced
¼   cup chopped raw walnuts
½   tsp. ground cinnamon
1   tsp. raw honey (optional)

- Combine almond milk, water, and quinoa in a medium saucepan and bring to a boil. Reduce heat to between low and medium. Cover and simmer until most of the liquid is absorbed, 12 to 14 minutes.

- Stir in the butter. Remove from the heat and let stand for about 5 minutes.
- Add the blueberries, strawberries, walnuts, and cinnamon and mix well. Drizzle with the honey if using.

Makes 4 servings.

Per serving: 270 calories, 12 g fat (7.5 g saturated), 32 g carbohydrates, 5.5 g sugars, 7 g protein, 5 g fiber

Eggs Florentine with Sun-Dried Tomato Pesto

1	tsp. olive oil
1	package (9 oz.) pre-washed spinach
⅓	cup fat-free Greek-style yogurt
¼	cup sun-dried tomato pesto
1	tsp. vinegar
	Pinch of salt
4	large eggs
2	whole-grain English muffins, split and toasted
	Fresh ground black pepper to taste

- Heat the olive oil in a nonstick skillet over medium-high heat. Sauté the spinach until wilted.
- Mix the yogurt and pesto in a small bowl and stir ¼ cup into the spinach. Remove from the heat and cover.
- Heat a medium saucepan with about an inch of water and bring to a boil. Add the vinegar and salt. Reduce the heat to low. Break an egg into a small teacup and tip the egg into the water. Do the same with the rest of the eggs. Cover and simmer until the eggs are soft-cooked.
- Place a toasted English muffin half on each of four plates. Spoon ¼ of the spinach onto each half. Remove the eggs with a slotted spoon to drain, and then place on top of the spinach.
- Spoon the yogurt and pesto sauce over each egg. Add pepper to taste.

Makes 4 servings.

Per serving: 175 calories, 6 g fat (2 g saturated), 21 g carbohydrates, 12 g protein, 5 g fiber

Huevos Rancheros

4 Tbsp. olive oil, divided
4 6" stone-ground corn tortillas
1 cup Amy's Organic Refried Black Beans, divided
6 oz. baby spinach
⅛ tsp. cayenne pepper
4 large eggs
1 large avocado, pitted, peeled, chopped, divided
4 Tbsp. crumbled queso fresco, divided
1 Tbsp. chopped cilantro, divided
  Salt and pepper, to taste
  Cholula Original Hot Sauce, to taste

- In a 12-inch nonstick skillet over medium-high heat, add 1 tablespoon olive oil. When the oil is hot, quickly sauté two tortillas until crispy on both sides. Repeat with the remaining tortillas. Place 2 tortillas on each plate.

- Spread ¼ cup of refried black beans over each tortilla.

- In the same skillet, add another tablespoon of olive oil, the baby spinach, and the cayenne. Sauté the greens until the leaves are wilted. Divide the spinach and top each tortilla with some.

- Reduce the heat to medium. In the same skillet, add the remaining 2 tablespoons of olive oil. Gently crack the eggs into the pan.

- Cover with a lid and cook the eggs until the whites are completely set but the yolks are still soft. Using a spatula, place an egg on each tortilla.

- Top off each plate with half the chopped avocado, 2 tablespoons of queso fresco, ½ tablespoon of cilantro, and salt, pepper, and hot sauce.

Makes 2 servings.

Per serving: 311 calories, 18 g fat (3 g saturated), 24 g carbohydrates, 15 g protein, 4 g fiber

Huevos Sedona

2   flaxseed wraps
2   cups fresh spinach leaves
¼   cup white onion, chopped
2   cloves garlic, chopped
2   tsp. grapeseed oil
1   cup canned black beans, rinsed
½   tsp. chili powder
½   tsp. cumin
¼   tsp. sea salt
¼   tsp. black pepper
8   egg whites
½   cup fresh salsa
½   avocado, sliced
1   Tbsp. cilantro, chopped

- Warm the wraps and top with spinach leaves. Place the wraps on dinner plates.

- Sauté the onion and garlic in 1 teaspoon of grapeseed oil for 1 minute. Add the black beans, chili powder, cumin, salt, and pepper. Cook for about 3 minutes, then move to a bowl and cover to keep warm.

- Add the remaining oil to the pan and scramble the egg whites in the pan over medium heat.

- Divide the bean mixture evenly and place over the spinach on each tortilla. Top with salsa, avocado, and cilantro.

Makes 2 servings.

Per serving: 323 calories, 11 g fat (1.5 g saturated), 34 carbohydrates, 5 g sugars, 25 g protein, 11 g fiber

Oatmeal & Berries

4½ cups water
1 cup steel-cut oats
½ cup oat bran
½ tsp. salt
18 walnut halves
2 large strawberries, sliced

- Mix the water, oats, oat bran, and salt in a medium saucepan.
- Bring to a boil over medium-high heat. Reduce the heat and cover the pan. Simmer, stirring frequently, until thickened.
- Serve topped with walnuts and strawberries.

Makes three 1-cup servings.

Per serving: 220 calories, 11 g fat (1.5 g saturated), 31 g carbohydrates, 8 g protein, 6 g fiber

Spinach & Cheese Omelet

2 eggs
1 slice Canadian bacon, diced
⅓ cup baby spinach leaves, chopped
Cooking spray
1 Tbsp. reduced-fat mozzarella cheese, shredded

- Whisk the eggs in a bowl and then add the diced bacon and spinach.
- Coat a skillet with cooking spray. Pour in the egg mixture and cook over medium heat until set.
- Flip the omelet, add the cheese, and fold the omelet in half.

Makes 1 serving.

Per serving: 200 calories, 12 g fat (4.5 g saturated), 20 g carbohydrates, 20 g protein, 0 g fiber

Get the Scoop

Protein powders aren't just for smoothies. Use them to add more nutrition to your foods.

1) **MAKE A FANCY PARFAIT.** Combine a small scoop of vanilla protein powder, plain Greek yogurt, mixed berries, cinnamon, and a handful of shaved almonds and get a flavorful treat any time of the day.

2) **SEW YOUR OATS.** Mix ¼ cup of steel-cut oats with 1 cup of water (or your favorite nut milk), 1 small scoop of protein powder, ½ tablespoon of flaxseed, a diced green apple, and nutmeg. Bring the water to a boil, add the oats, reduce the heat to low, and let simmer for 30 minutes. Add in all your fixings at the end to get a perfectly warm bowl of healthy oats or chilled overnight oats.

3) **MUSCLE UP BROWNIES.** Add protein powder to your cookie, brownie, and cake batter.

Snacks

Devilishly Good Eggs

6   eggs
1   Tbsp. extra-virgin olive oil
1½ Tbsp. pickle relish
½   tsp. hot paprika
    Pinch sea salt

- Place the eggs in a saucepan and cover with cold water until there's about 1½ inches of water above the eggs. Bring the water to a boil, then cover and reduce the heat to low and cook for 1 minute. Remove from heat and leave covered for 15 minutes, then rinse under cold water for 1 minute.

- Crack the eggshells and carefully peel the eggs under cool running water. Gently dry with paper towels. Slice the eggs in half lengthwise, removing yolks. Place the yolks in a bowl, the whites on a serving platter. Mash the yolks with a fork, then mix in the olive oil, relish, paprika, and salt. Mash some more. Add a scoop of the egg mixture to each egg white half, sprinkle with a little more paprika, and either serve or refrigerate. The eggs will be fresh for five days.

Makes 6 servings (2 halves).

Per serving: 84 calories, 6.6 g fat (2.3 g saturated), 5.6 g protein

Fruit Salad with Lime and Mint

3   cups honeydew melon balls
1   cup blueberries
1   cup blackberries
1½ Tbsp. chopped fresh mint
1   Tbsp. fresh lime juice

- Place the melon balls, berries, mint, and lime juice in a mixing bowl and toss to combine. Serve in martini glasses.

Makes 4 servings.

Per serving: 90 calories, 0 g fat, 23 g carbohydrates, 1 g protein, 3 g fiber

Guacamole

2   ripe avocados, peeled and pitted
¼   cup finely chopped red onion
2   Tbsp. fresh cilantro, chopped
1   Tbsp. fresh lime juice
½   ripe tomato, seeded and diced
½   tsp. sea salt

- Mash the avocado with a fork in a medium bowl.
- Add the rest of the ingredients and mix well. Refrigerate.

Makes sixteen 2-Tbsp. servings.

Per serving: 61 calories, 5.3 g fat (0.7 g saturated), 3.9 g carbohydrates, 0.6 g sugars, 0.8 g protein, 2.5 g fiber

Melon Slush

5   ice cubes
4   cups cubed cantaloupe
1½ tsp. fresh lemon juice
1½ tsp. stevia (optional)

- Place the ice cubes in a blender and blend until just crushed. Add the cantaloupe, lemon juice, and stevia. Blend on high.

Makes 4 servings.

Per serving: 60 calories, 0 g fat, 13 g carbohydrates, 1 g protein, 1 g fiber

More Quick Snacks
12 fast and easy ways to crush a craving

If you need a little something to take the edge off hunger, avoid high-carb snacks like chips, pretzels, cake, or ice cream. Go for a combo of protein and carbohydrate to stabilize your blood sugar and satisfy your belly. Here are some easy ideas:

- 10 Goldfish crackers and ½ cup skim milk.

- String cheese and whole-grain crackers.

- 1 cup of popcorn and ½ cup skim milk.

- Five baby carrots with chickpea hummus.

- Jicama triangles with a dollop of guacamole.

- Celery sticks with a tablespoon of peanut butter.

- A small bowl of oatmeal or whole-grain, low-sugar cereal with milk.

- ¼ cup cottage cheese and ½ cup strawberries, blueberries, raspberries, or blackberries.

- Apple slices with almond butter.

- Slice of turkey breast deli meat rolled up with a slice of Swiss cheese.

- Strawberries dipped in melted dark chocolate.

- Cucumber shooters. Take a 2- to 3-inch-thick slice of large cucumber, scoop out the seeds, and fill the veggie "shot glass" with hummus or tzatziki. Eat as is or use carrot sticks for dipping.

Lunches

Avocado Salad

2   Tbsp. extra-virgin olive oil
1½   Tbsp. fresh lime juice
2   tsp. honey
¼   tsp. kosher salt
⅛   tsp. ground red pepper
1   romaine lettuce head, chopped (about 3 cups)
1   cup thinly sliced radishes (5 medium)
1   ripe avocado, diced

• Combine the first 5 ingredients in a large bowl. Add the remaining
  ingredients, and toss.

Makes 4 servings.

Per serving: 143 calories, 12.4 g fat (1.7 g saturated), 8 g carbohydrates,
4 g sugars, 1 g protein, 4 g fiber

Black Bean Salad with Avocado

2   cups chopped romaine lettuce hearts
1   medium avocado, chopped into bite-size pieces
1   medium tomato, chopped into bite-size pieces
½   cup canned black beans, rinsed and drained
2   Tbsp. diced green onion
1   Tbsp. diced fresh cilantro
1   Tbsp. olive oil
2   tsp. lime juice
½   tsp. lime zest
¼   tsp. salt
½   tsp. ground black pepper

• Toss the lettuce, avocado, tomato, beans, green onion, and cilantro
  in a large salad bowl.

• In a small bowl, stir the olive oil, lime juice, lime zest, salt, and pepper.
  Pour over the salad, and toss to coat.

Makes 2 servings.

Per serving: 247 calories, 17 g fat (2 g saturated), 20 g carbohydrates, 3 g sugars, 6 g protein, 9 g fiber

Chicken Salad Roll-Ups

2   chicken breasts, cooked and chopped
½   cup celery, diced
½   scallion, diced
2   Tbsp. light mayonnaise
     Salt and pepper
½   cup halved seedless red grapes
2   romaine or red lettuce leaves

- Mix the chicken, celery, scallion and mayonnaise in a bowl, and season with salt and pepper. Gently stir in the grapes.
- Divide between the lettuce and roll up.

Makes 2 servings.

Per serving: 230 calories, 8 g fat (1.5 g saturated), 10 g carbohydrates, 27 g protein, 1 g fiber

Wrap It in Greens

Boston, butter, Bibb, and other soft lettuce leaves are terrific substitutes for bread in sandwiches. Take a large lettuce leaf and fill it with egg salad, tuna salad, chicken salad, or hummus and roll it into a handheld meal. Or snack. Slip them into a zip-lock plastic bag to go.

Cream of Tomato Soup

1 Tbsp. extra-virgin olive oil
1 small onion, chopped
2 cups vegetable or chicken broth
1 can (14 oz.) diced tomatoes
2 Tbsp. tomato paste
1 tsp. dried basil, crushed
1 cup half-and-half or canned coconut milk
¼ cup fresh basil, chopped

• In a large saucepan over medium-high heat, heat the olive oil. Cook the onion, stirring occasionally, for 5 minutes, or until soft. Add the broth, tomatoes (with juice), tomato paste, and dried basil. Bring to a boil. Reduce the heat to low, cover, and simmer for 20 minutes, or until slightly thickened. Let cool for 10 minutes.

• Transfer the mixture in batches to a blender or food processor. Puree until smooth. Return to the saucepan. Add the half-and-half. Cook, stirring, for 3 minutes, or until heated and thickened. Serve garnished with the fresh basil.

Makes 4 servings.

Per serving: 153 calories, 10 g fat (5 g saturated), 12 g carbohydrates, 3 g protein, 2 g fiber

Greek Salad

5 cups washed ready-to-eat salad
8 cherry tomatoes
½ cup radishes, trimmed and cut into quarters
2 Tbsp. reduced-fat oil and vinegar dressing
1 Tbsp. crumbled feta cheese

• Place the salad in a bowl. Add the tomatoes and radishes.

• Add the dressing and toss.

• Sprinkle the feta cheese on top and serve.

Makes 2 servings.

Per serving: 64 calories, 2.5 g fat (0.9 g saturated), 13 g carbohydrates, 5.0 g sugars, 3.2 g protein, 4.1 g fiber

Portobello Turkey Burger & Bruschetta

8 oz. ground turkey
½ tsp. garlic powder
¼ tsp. kosher salt
¼ tsp. black pepper
Olive oil for greasing the grill
4 large portobello mushroom caps (stems removed)
2 Tbsp. balsamic vinegar
1 Tbsp. red onion, chopped
2 fresh basil leaves, sliced thinly
2 plum tomatoes, chopped
1 oz. mozzarella, sliced

- In a bowl, mix the turkey, garlic powder, salt, and pepper. Form burger patties.
- Lightly oil a grill or grill pan and heat to medium-high heat.
- Cook the burgers and mushroom caps, about 4 minutes per side, until burger is cooked and the portobellos are tender.
- Mix the vinegar, onion, basil, and tomato. Add salt and pepper to taste.
- Place each burger on a mushroom cap, top with a mozzarella slice and bruschetta mixture, and use the remaining mushrooms as "bun" tops.

Makes 2 servings.

Per serving: 260 calories, 12 g fat (3.5 g saturated), 13 g carbohydrates, 9 g sugars, 30 g protein, 3 g fiber

Roast Beef and Horseradish Wrap

2   tsp. light mayonnaise
½   tsp. prepared horseradish
1   whole-wheat tortilla
1   large romaine lettuce leaf
3   slices lean roast beef
¼   cup chopped tomato

- Mix the mayonnaise and horseradish in a small bowl. Spread the mixture on one side of the tortilla.

- Place the lettuce leaf in the center of the tortilla, followed by roast beef and tomato. Fold the outer edges in, and then roll.

Makes 1 serving.

Per serving: 190 calories, 6 g fat (1.5 saturated), 23 g carbohydrates, 17 g protein, 3 g fiber

Strawberry Pecan Salad

2   Tbsp. balsamic vinegar
1   tsp. raw honey
¼   cup olive oil
      Salt to taste
3   cups baby spinach
1   cup strawberries, sliced
¼   cup pecan halves

- Mix the balsamic vinegar and honey in a bowl.

- Whisk in the olive oil. Add salt as desired.

- Divide the spinach on four plates. Top with strawberries and pecans. Drizzle balsamic vinaigrette on top.

Makes 4 servings.

Per serving: 176 calories, 16 g fat (3 g saturated), 9 g carbohydrates, 3 g sugars, 2 g protein, 3 g fiber

Tex-Mex Bean Salad

1   can (15 oz.) pinto beans, rinsed and drained
1   can chickpeas, rinsed and drained
1   can (14.5 oz.) Mexican-style diced tomatoes
1   can corn
1   onion, chopped
1   red bell pepper, chopped
½   cup carrots, chopped
3   garlic cloves, minced
2   Tbsp. red wine vinegar
½   cup olive oil
½   tsp. chili powder
¼   tsp. ground red pepper

- Add the beans, chickpeas, tomatoes, corn, onion, bell pepper, carrots, and garlic to a large bowl and mix.
- Add the vinegar, oil, chili powder, and ground red pepper. Mix to coat evenly.
- Let stand in a refrigerator for 30 minutes, mixing twice.

Makes 8 servings.

Per serving: 136 calories, 3 g fat (0 g saturated), 22 g carbohydrates, 5 g protein, 5 g fiber

Watermelon Salad with Yogurt

2   cups 2% Greek yogurt
2   Tbsp. lemon juice
2   Tbsp. dill, chopped
2   Tbsp. mint, chopped
½   tsp. kosher salt
½   tsp. black pepper
1   cup cucumber, chopped
1   cup seedless watermelon, chopped
1   cup grape tomatoes, halved
2   Tbsp. red onion, diced
2   Tbsp. roasted, salted pistachios, shelled

- Whisk the yogurt, lemon juice, dill, mint, salt, and pepper.
- In a bowl, combine the cucumber, watermelon, tomatoes, and onion.
- Mix in yogurt sauce until well combined. Refrigerate until serving. Top each serving with pistachios.

Makes 2 servings.

Per serving: 186 calories, 6 g fat (2 g saturated), 23 g carbohydrates, 14 g sugars, 13 g protein, 3 g fiber

Dinners

Beef Stew

¼ cup all-purpose flour
1 tsp. salt, plus more to taste
½ tsp. freshly ground black pepper, plus more to taste
1½ pounds lean stewing beef cut into 1½" cubes
2 Tbsp. vegetable oil
2 onions, chopped
3 cloves garlic, minced
1 tsp. dried marjoram
1 tsp. dried thyme
1 bay leaf
1 cup red wine
3 Tbsp. tomato paste
3 cups reduced-sodium beef broth
5 large carrots
2 stalks celery
5 potatoes (about 1½ pounds)
12 oz. fresh green beans
⅓ cup chopped fresh parsley

- Combine the flour, salt, and pepper, and beef in a large zip-top plastic bag and shake to coat. Transfer to a plate and save the leftover flour mixture.

- In a Dutch oven, heat 1 tablespoon of vegetable oil over medium heat. Add the beef in batches, adding more oil as needed during cooking until the meat is browned all around. Transfer each batch to a plate when finished.

- Reduce the heat to medium-low. Add the onions, garlic, marjoram, thyme, bay leaf, and the rest of the flour mixture to the pan. Cook, stirring often, until the onions are soft, about 4 minutes. Add the red wine and tomato paste to the pan and stir with a wooden spoon.

- Put the beef back into the pan along with the broth. Bring to a boil, stirring often, until slightly thickened. Reduce the heat to medium low, cover, and simmer for an hour, stirring occasionally.

- Cut the carrots and celery into 1½-inch pieces. Peel and quarter the potatoes. After the stew has cooked for an hour, add the vegetables to the Dutch oven. Cover and simmer for 30 minutes.

- Trim the ends of the beans and cut in half. Add the beans to the pan and stir. Cover and simmer for 30 more minutes. Remove the bay leaf and add the parsley. Season with salt and pepper to taste.

Makes 6 servings.

Per serving: 362 calories, 12 g fat (3 g saturated), 35 g carbohydrates, 27 g protein, 5 g fiber

Chicken Chili

2½ lbs. boneless, skinless chicken breasts
2   medium onions, chopped
2   cloves garlic, minced
1   Tbsp. olive oil
4   cans cannellini beans (15.5 oz. each), rinsed and drained
2   cans (14 oz. each) fat-free, reduced-sodium chicken broth
1   can (4.5 oz.) chopped green chilies
1   tsp. salt
1   tsp. ground cumin
¾ tsp. dried oregano
½ tsp. chili powder
½ tsp. ground black pepper
⅛ tsp. ground cloves
⅛ tsp. ground red pepper

- Cut the chicken breasts into bite-size chunks, then sauté with onions and garlic in a Dutch oven in the olive oil heated over medium-high heat.
- When the chicken is browned, add the beans, broth, chilies, salt, and spices.
- Bring to a boil, then reduce the heat and simmer uncovered for 35 minutes.

Makes 10 servings.

Per serving: 230 calories, 4 g fat (1 g saturated), 12 g carbohydrates, 35 g protein, 4 g fiber

Chicken Gumbo

3   Tbsp. vegetable oil
1   small onion
3   celery ribs, chopped
1   large green bell pepper, chopped
1   garlic clove, minced
½   tsp. ground black pepper
3½   Tbsp. whole-wheat flour
2½– 3 cans (14 ½ oz. each) reduced-sodium chicken broth
¾   cup crushed tomatoes
¼   lb. boneless smoked ham, cut into ½" pieces
3   skinless chicken thighs (¾ lb.)
1   tsp. dried thyme
1   bay leaf
⅛   tsp. ground red pepper
1   Tbsp. chopped fresh parsley

- Heat the vegetable oil in a soup pot over medium heat.
- Add the onion, celery, bell pepper, garlic, and black pepper.
- Cover and cook just until the vegetables begin to soften, 5 to 6 minutes.
- Stir in the flour and cook, stirring frequently, for 3 minutes.
- Gradually stir in 2½ cans of the broth and bring it to a simmer.
- Add the tomatoes, ham, chicken, thyme, bay leaf, and ground red pepper.
- Partially cover, and cook until the chicken is tender, 25 to 35 minutes, adding the remaining broth as necessary if the gumbo is too thick.
- Remove from the heat, transfer the chicken to a plate, and let cool slightly.
- Cut into bite-size pieces, discarding the bones, and return to the pot.
- Reheat briefly and stir in the parsley.
- Remove the bay leaf before serving.

Makes 6 servings.

Per serving: 214 calories, 12 g fat (2 g saturated), 10 g carbohydrates, 13 g protein, 2 g fiber

Chicken Parmesan

Sauce

1	Tbsp. olive oil
2	garlic cloves, minced
1¼	cups canned crushed tomatoes
2	Tbsp. Italian-style tomato paste
¼	cup chopped fresh basil
¼	tsp. dried oregano
¼	tsp. salt
¼	tsp. ground black pepper

Chicken

6	slices light whole-wheat bread
2	large eggs
2	Tbsp. water
4	boneless, skinless chicken breast halves (6 oz. each), pounded to ¼" thickness
¼	tsp. salt
½	tsp. ground black pepper
¼	cup soy flour or whole-wheat flour
2	tsp. olive oil
6	oz. shredded part-skim mozzarella cheese

TO MAKE THE SAUCE:

- Heat the olive oil in a small saucepan over low heat.
- Stir in the garlic and cook, stirring frequently, for 30 seconds.
- Add the tomatoes, tomato paste, oregano, and basil.
- Cook until thick and rich, 12 to 15 minutes, stirring occasionally.
- Season with the salt and pepper.
- Cover and keep warm.

TO MAKE THE CHICKEN:

- While the sauce is cooking, preheat the oven to 250°F.
- Place the bread on a rimmed baking sheet and bake until completely dry, 10 to 12 minutes.
- Let cool slightly.

134

- Transfer the bread to a food processor and grind to make about 1 cup crumbs.
- Remove to a large plate.
- In a shallow bowl, lightly beat the eggs with the water.
- Season the chicken with salt and pepper and coat with the flour.
- Dip into the egg mixture, then press the crumbs to coat both sides.
- Place the broiler rack 4 to 5 inches from the heat and preheat the broiler.
- Heat 1 teaspoon of the olive oil in a large skillet over medium heat.
- Add 2 of the coated chicken breasts and cook until golden brown on the first side, 2 to 3 minutes.
- Turn and cook until no longer pink and the juices run clear, 2 to 3 minutes.
- Remove to a 13 x 9-inch baking dish.
- Repeat with the remaining teaspoon of oil and remaining chicken.
- Top with the sauce and sprinkle with the cheese.
- Broil just until the cheese melts, 1 to 2 minutes.

Makes 6 servings.

Per serving: 361 calories, 18 g fat (3 g saturated), 16 g carbohydrates, 29 g protein, 3 g fiber

Kale & Cannellini Beans

2   tsp. extra-virgin olive oil, plus more if desired
1   large clove garlic, minced
1   large bunch kale, chopped
1   can (15 oz.) cannellini beans, drained and rinsed
    Sea salt and cracked black pepper

- Heat the olive oil in a large skillet over medium heat. Add the garlic and cook for 1 minute. Add the kale and sauté until wilted, 3 to 4 minutes. Add the beans and heat through. Season with salt and pepper. If desired, drizzle a bit more oil over the greens.

Makes 6 servings.

Per serving: 110 calories, 2.5 g fat (0 g saturated), 18 g carbohydrates, 5 g protein, 4 g fiber

Chicken & Vegetable Kebabs with Quinoa

1   lb. boneless chicken breast, cut into 1-inch cubes
½   cup teriyaki sauce
1   medium onion, cut into 1-inch pieces
1   red bell pepper, cut into 1-inch pieces
2   zucchinis, cut into ½-inch pieces
½   cup cooked quinoa

- Marinate the chicken cubes in teriyaki sauce in the refrigerator for 30 minutes or longer. Place 8 wooden skewers in a pan of water while the chicken is marinating.
- Divide the chicken, onion, bell pepper, and zucchini chunks evenly on the skewers.
- Brush with the remaining marinade.
- Heat a grill to medium heat, and grill the skewers, turning frequently until cooked through, about 12 minutes.
- Place two cooked skewers over quinoa on each plate to serve.

Makes 4 servings.

Per serving: 461 calories, 6 g fat (2.5 g saturated), 18.6 g carbohydrates, 39.9 g protein, 12.6 g fiber

Cod with Romesco Sauce

For the cod:

2   Tbsp. olive oil
4   skinless cod fillets (5 oz. each)
2   tsp. chopped fresh chives
½   tsp. sea salt
¼   tsp. ground black pepper
½   of the yield of romesco sauce

- In a large nonstick skillet over medium-high heat, heat the olive oil. Sprinkle the cod with the chives, salt, and pepper. Cook for 8 minutes, turning once, or until the fish flakes easily. Remove to a plate.
- Add the romesco sauce to the skillet, reduce the heat to medium, and bring to a boil. Cook, stirring, for 1 minute, or until heated through. Pour over the cod.

Makes 4 servings.

Per serving: 234 calories, 12 g total fat (2 g saturated), 3 g carbohydrates, 27 g protein, 1 g fiber

For the romesco sauce:

2   Tbsp. extra-virgin olive oil
¼   cup slivered almonds
4   cloves garlic, coarsely chopped
¼   tsp. red pepper flakes
1   can fire-roasted tomatoes
¼   cup pimientos, drained
2   Tbsp. ground golden flaxseeds
2   Tbsp. red wine vinegar
½   tsp. sea salt

- In a small skillet over medium-high heat, heat 1 tablespoon of the olive oil. Cook the almonds, garlic, and pepper flakes, stirring, for 3 minutes, or until the almonds are lightly roasted. Transfer the almond mixture to a food processor along with the tomatoes, pimientos, flaxseeds, vinegar, salt, and the remaining 1 tablespoon oil. Process until well combined and smooth.

- Store in an airtight container in the refrigerator for up to 2 weeks or in the freezer for up to 3 months.

Makes 16 servings (2 cups).

Per serving (2 Tbsp.): 57 calories, 5 g fat (0.5 g saturated), 3 g carbohydrates, 2 g protein, 1 g fiber

Diner-Style Meatloaf

2   Tbsp. olive or coconut oil, plus more for greasing the baking sheet
1   small onion, finely chopped
1   carrot, finely chopped
1   rib celery, finely chopped
2   cloves garlic, minced
2   pounds ground beef
¼   cup ground flaxseeds
2   large eggs
½   cup tomato juice
2   Tbsp. chopped fresh parsley
1   tsp. sea salt
½   tsp. ground black pepper
4   strips bacon, cut in half

- Preheat the oven to 350°F.
- Lightly oil a rimmed baking sheet.
- In a large skillet over medium heat, heat the olive oil. Cook the onion, carrot, celery, and garlic, stirring occasionally, for 5 minutes, or until tender. Transfer to a large bowl and let cool to room temperature.
- Add the beef, flaxseeds, eggs, tomato juice, parsley, salt, and pepper to the bowl. Mix thoroughly.
- With your hands, transfer the mixture to the baking sheet and shape into a log about 9 x 5 inches. Lay the bacon strips lengthwise over the top and sides. Press to adhere. Bake for 1 hour 15 minutes, or until a thermometer inserted in the center registers 160°F and the meat is no longer pink. Let rest for 10 minutes before slicing.

Makes 8 servings.

Per serving: 386 calories, 20 g fat (7 g saturated), 24 g carbohydrates, 27 g protein, 2 g fiber

Eggplant Parmesan

2	eggplants (2 lbs. each), peeled and sliced lengthwise into slabs ¼" thick
3	Tbsp. olive oil
½	tsp. salt
1	can (15½ oz.) crushed or chopped tomatoes (with juice)
1	Tbsp. + 1 ½ tsp. tomato paste
1	tsp. dried basil or 3 large fresh basil leaves, chopped
½	tsp. dried rosemary, crumbled
¼	tsp. ground black pepper
1	cup (4 oz.) shredded mozzarella or Fontina cheese
½	cup (2 oz.) grated Parmesan cheese

- Preheat the broiler. Place the eggplant on a large rimmed baking sheet and brush both sides with the olive oil (work in batches if necessary). Sprinkle with ¼ teaspoon of the salt.
- Broil 5" from the heat until just beginning to brown, 2 to 3 minutes per side.
- Set the oven temperature to 375°F.
- In a saucepan, combine the tomatoes (with juice), tomato paste, basil, and rosemary. Cook over medium-low heat, stirring occasionally, until slightly thickened, about 15 minutes. Season with the remaining ¼ teaspoon salt and the pepper.

- Spread a layer of the tomato mixture over the bottom of a 1 ½-quart baking dish. Add a layer of eggplant and top with another layer of the tomato mixture. Sprinkle with a thin layer of the mozzarella and the Parmesan.
- Continue making 2 more layers with the remaining eggplant, tomato mixture, and cheeses, ending with a thick layer of cheeses.
- Bake until bubbling, 25 to 30 minutes.
- Let rest for 10 minutes before cutting.

Makes 6 servings.

Per serving: 224 calories, 14 g fat (5 g saturated), 16 g carbohydrates, 11 g protein, 5 g fiber

Flank Steak Salad

1   plum tomato, cut in eighths
¼   cup sliced onion
1   small clove garlic, crushed
2½   cups chopped romaine lettuce
2   Tbsp. balsamic vinaigrette
      Salt and pepper
      Grilled flank steak slices
2   Tbsp. crumbled blue cheese

- Mix the tomato, onion, garlic, and lettuce in a bowl. Add the vinaigrette and toss to coat. Season with salt and pepper.
- Top with grilled steak and cheese.

Makes 1 serving.

Per serving: 350 calories, 16 g fat (7 g saturated), 16 g carbohydrates, 38 g protein, 4 g fiber

Pesto Chicken Sandwich

4   whole-wheat tortillas (6" diameter)
¼   cup jarred pesto sauce
½   pound sliced cooked chicken breast, warmed
¼   tsp. salt
¼   tsp. ground black pepper
2   jarred roasted red bell peppers (2 oz.), drained and halved
4   thin slices (3 to 4 oz.) mozzarella cheese
4   romaine lettuce leaves

- Preheat the oven to 350°F. Arrange the tortillas on a rimmed baking sheet.
- Spread the pesto evenly over each tortilla.
- Arrange the chicken in a row down the center of each tortilla and sprinkle with the salt and black pepper.
- Top with the roasted peppers and mozzarella.
- Bake just until heated through and the cheese melts.
- Top with lettuce, roll into a cylinder, and serve.

Makes 4 servings.

Per serving: 328 calories, 16 g fat (6 g saturated), 23 g carbohydrates, 29 g protein, 3 g fiber

Planked Salmon with Grilled Asparagus and Roasted New Potatoes

2   wild-caught salmon fillets (for four 4-oz. servings)
    Salt and pepper
4   Tbsp. grainy mustard
6   Tbsp. packed brown sugar

- Soak 2 cedar planks in cold water for at least an hour. Remove and dry.
- Rinse the salmon under cold water and pat dry with paper towels.
- Season the flesh side of the fillets with salt and pepper. Using a brush, spread the mustard over the fish. Crush the brown sugar in a bowl with a fork, then sprinkle over the fillets.
- Place the cedar planks on a medium-hot grill for 3 minutes, until you can smell smoke. Then turn the planks over and place the coated fillets on the planks skin-side down. Cover the grill and cook the fish for about 20 minutes or until the fish is cooked through. If your plank edges begin to flame, mist them with a spray bottle of water. When done, serve from the plank.

Grilled asparagus

8   oz. asparagus, tough ends trimmed
1½   Tbsp. extra-virgin olive oil
     Sea salt and cracked black pepper

- Brush the asparagus with oil and grill, turning until tender, 7 minutes.

New potatoes

1   lb. small new potatoes, cubed
2   Tbsp. lemon juice
1   Tbsp. olive oil
¼   cup chopped fresh oregano
¼   tsp. salt
¼   tsp. ground black pepper

- Preheat the oven to 425°F.
- Place the potatoes in a bowl, sprinkle with the lemon juice, and toss.
- Coat a 13 x 9-inch baking pan with the oil and spread the potatoes on the pan in one layer. Bake for 15 minutes.
- Turn the potatoes with a spatula and mist with no-stick spray. Bake for 20 minutes.
- Spray again and toss with the oregano. Bake for another 5 minutes, or until the potatoes are browned on the outside. Sprinkle with the salt and pepper.

Makes 4 servings.

Per serving: 441 calories, 22 g fat (2.5 g saturated), 46 g carbohydrates, 35 g protein, 5 g fiber

Roasted Brussels Sprouts

2   Tbsp. coconut oil
2   leeks, white parts only, cut in rounds
1½ lbs. Brussels sprouts, halved
     Coarse sea salt and pepper to taste

- Heat the coconut oil in a skillet over medium heat.
- Sauté the leeks in a large saucepan for 2 minutes.
- Add the Brussels sprouts and cook for 7 minutes, stirring often, until roasted on the outside. Season with sea salt and pepper.

Makes 6 servings.

Per serving: 106 calories, 5 g fat (4 g saturated), 7 g carbohydrates, 4 g protein, 5 g fiber

Salmon Burger with Dill

Canola oil spray
2   6-oz. cans salmon, drained
1   small onion, finely chopped
1   egg
⅓   cup bread crumbs
¼   cup light mayonnaise
2   tsp. dried dill
2   Tbsp. fat-free Greek yogurt
1   tsp. Dijon mustard
4   whole-wheat rolls
4   leaves romaine lettuce
4   tomato slices

- Preheat the oven to 350°F. Coat a rimmed baking sheet with canola oil spray.

- Mix the salmon, onion, egg, bread crumbs, mayonnaise, and dill well in a bowl and form into 4 even patties.

- Put the patties on the baking sheet and bake flipping once halfway through the baking time, until browned.

- Mix the yogurt and mustard in a bowl. Divide the sauce evenly and spread it on the rolls. Add the burgers to the rolls and top with lettuce and tomatoes.

Makes 4 servings.

Per serving: 320 calories, 11 g fat (2 g saturated), 720 mg sodium, 29 g carbohydrates, 25 g protein, 4 g fiber

Shrimp & Clams Stew

1   Tbsp. olive oil
½   cup onion, chopped
½   cup red bell pepper, chopped
1   clove garlic, minced
1   can (28 oz.) diced tomatoes (with juice)
1   can (28 oz.) tomato sauce
¼   cup dry red wine
¼   cup fresh parsley, chopped
1   tsp. Worcestershire sauce
½   tsp. dried oregano
1   tsp. red pepper flakes
8   oz. bay scallops
8   oz. medium wild-caught shrimp, peeled and deveined
1   can (10 oz.) whole baby clams
1   package baby spinach

- Heat the olive oil in a Dutch oven over medium-high heat. Add the
  onion, bell pepper, and garlic. Sauté for 5 minutes or until the onion is
  tender.

- Add the tomatoes (with juice), tomato sauce, wine, parsley,
  Worcestershire, oregano, and pepper flakes. Stir well. Bring to a boil
  over medium heat, then simmer, covered, for 20 minutes, stirring
  occasionally.

- Add the scallops, shrimp, and clams. Bring to a boil. Stir. Reduce the
  heat and simmer for 8 minutes or until the scallops are tender and
  the shrimp turn pink. During the last minute of cooking, add the baby
  spinach.

Makes 6 servings.

Per serving: 288 calories, 5 g fat (1 g saturated), 22 g carbohydrates,
37 g protein, 4.5 g fiber

Tequila Sunrise Salad

For the salad:

2½ cups mixed greens
¼ cup black beans, rinsed and drained
1 plum tomato, chopped
1 scallion, chopped
½ avocado, peeled and sliced
1 tsp. fresh cilantro, chopped

For the dressing:

1 Tbsp. tequila
1 Tbsp. orange juice
1 tsp. lime juice
1 tsp. extra-virgin olive oil
   Cracked black pepper

- Mix the salad ingredients in a bowl. Mix the dressing in another bowl and pour over the salad. Toss to coat.

Makes 1 serving.

Per serving: 325 calories, 21 g fat (3 g saturated), 22 g carbohydrates, 8 g protein, 13 g fiber

Tuna Salad Wrapped in Lettuce

2 cans (6 oz. each) water-packed tuna, drained
¼ cup mayonnaise
1 tsp. Dijon mustard
1 Tbsp. lemon juice
2 Tbsp. red bell pepper, finely chopped
2 Tbsp. celery, finely chopped
2 tsp. capers, drained
2 scallions, thinly sliced
¼ tsp. salt
⅛ tsp. pepper
8 large Boston or butter lettuce leaves

- Flake the tuna in a medium bowl using a fork. Mix in the mayonnaise, mustard, and lemon juice.
- Add the bell pepper, celery, capers, scallions, salt, and pepper.

- One at a time, cup a lettuce leaf in the palm of your hand, spoon the tuna salad onto the leaf near the rib side, and roll to close.

Makes 4 servings.

Per serving: 157 calories, 6 g fat (1.5 g saturated), 2 g carbohydrates, 25 g protein, 1 g fiber

White Bean Soup with Sausage

1   Tbsp. + 1 tsp. olive oil
½   lb. sweet Italian sausage, casing removed, broken into 1" pieces
½   large onion, chopped
3   celery ribs, chopped
2½ cups chopped green or red cabbage
1   cup dried white beans, soaked overnight and drained
4–5 cans (14½ oz. each) reduced-sodium chicken broth
1   can (15 oz.) no-salt-added stewed tomatoes
1   tsp. dried Italian seasoning
1   large bay leaf
¼   tsp. ground black pepper

- Heat 1 teaspoon of the olive oil in a soup pot over medium-low heat.
- Add the sausage and cook, stirring occasionally, about 5 minutes.
- Remove to a plate, cover, and refrigerate.
- Pour the remaining olive oil into the same pot over medium heat.
- Stir in the onion, celery, and cabbage.
- Cook, stirring, until the vegetables begin to soften, 8 to 10 minutes.
- Add the beans, 4 cans of broth, and tomatoes to the pot. Bring to a boil and immediately reduce the heat, skimming off any froth.
- Stir in the Italian seasoning and bay leaf. Partially cover, and cook until the beans are tender, 1¼ to 1½ hours.
- Stir in the sausage and pepper. Simmer 2 minutes. Discard bay leaf.

Makes 8 servings.

Per serving: 218 calories, 13 g fat (4 g saturated), 17 g carbohydrates, 12 g protein, 5 g fiber

CHAPTER

10

Move More Every Day

The No Sugar Diet exercise plan

IF WE STILL toiled in the fields and factories, using our legs and arms to get our work done, as our grandparents and great-grandparents did, this chapter probably wouldn't be necessary. But today we sit a lot, way more than our ancestors did, and we walk much less. We plop our butts at our computers, in our cars, and on our couches. And as a result, most of us aren't burning off the calories we consume, and we gain weight and grow bigger bellies. Diabetes researchers estimate that for every inch your waist circumference expands, you increase your risk of type 2 diabetes by 8 percent.

You can do something pretty powerful to keep that from happening: Move more every day. Several large studies have shown that regular physical activity can have a big impact on your blood sugar. In one Finnish study, people who exercised for about 35 minutes a day dropped their risk of diabetes by 80 percent. That's huge! What's more, those people lowered risk even if they didn't lose any weight. That's because when you exercise, your body uses insulin more efficiently. Exercising boosts the number of insulin receptors on your cells, which helps insulin move blood sugar into cells where it can be used for fuel.

If you are currently sedentary, adding any kind of physical activity to your day is a step in the right direction. Choose something you like to do and you'll be more likely to stick to it.

However, for the next two weeks while on the 14-Day No Sugar Diet, I suggest you follow a structured routine that includes aerobic exercise and strength training. I'm including both because the combo punch appears to deliver a powerful blow to diabetes. Aerobic exercise helps insulin do a better job of lowering blood glucose, while strength training (also called resistance training) builds muscle, which provides more storage area for that glucose. Research reported in *PLOS Medicine* suggests that doing two and a half hours of cardio exercise and at least an hour of strength training per week can lower your risk of type 2 diabetes by two-thirds. That's actually very minimal exercise time over the course of a week, so anyone should be able to do it.

Picking up the pace in an aerobic workout seems to make a difference, too. Have you heard of interval training? It's nothing more than alternating between short bursts of fast, intense movement and slow-paced "rest" segments.

Think city driving versus highway driving. This is what an interval-walking workout looks like:

> **5-minute warm-up**	easy pace
> **1 minute**	fast pace
> **2 minutes**	moderate pace
> **1 minute**	fast pace
> **2 minutes**	moderate pace
> **1 minute**	fast pace
> **2 minutes**	moderate pace
> **1 minute**	fast pace
> **2 minutes**	moderate pace
> **1 minute**	fast pace
> **2 minutes**	moderate pace
> **1 minute**	fast pace
> **2 minutes**	moderate pace
> **1 minute**	fast pace
> **5-minute cool-down**	slow easy pace

One advantage of the speed-up/slow-down style of exercise is that it burns more calories than steady-pace exercise does in a shorter period of time. You get more bang for your buck, because it ensures that you truly exert yourself, not just go through the motions.

Another plus: High-Intensity Interval Training (HIIT) appears to help insulin do its job better. In a Scandinavian study, people with type 2 diabetes did either a moderately intense exercise program or an HIIT plan. After just six sessions over 14 days, the HIIT group improved insulin sensitivity much more than the lower-intensity exercise group did. In fact, the HIIT exercisers showed a return to normal glucose metabolism after just 2 weeks, suggesting that HIIT may actually work as effectively as diabetes medication.

For the No Sugar Diet exercise plan, you will be doing a mixture of HIIT walks, steady-pace walks, and resistance training. The workouts are described later in this chapter. Here's your exercise schedule for the next 14 days.

Your Move-More Schedule

Week 1

Monday	30-minute HIIT walk
Tuesday	Strength workout
Wednesday	30-minute HIIT walk
Thursday	Strength workout
Friday	30-minute HIIT walk
Saturday	The Big Burn 60-minute steady walk
Sunday	Rest

Week 2

Monday	Strength workout
Tuesday	30-minute HIIT walk
Wednesday	30-minute HIIT walk
Thursday	Strength workout
Friday	30-minute HIIT walk
Saturday	The Big Burn 60-minute steady walk
Sunday	Rest

Plus, do this every day: Enjoy a short, 15-minute stroll after dinner. Taking a walk within a half hour of eating will help you manage the post-meal surge of blood sugar.

14-Day No Sugar Diet High-Intensity Interval Training Walking Workout

How to do it:

• Wear a pair of supportive walking shoes or running shoes and clothing appropriate to the weather and activity that'll break a sweat.

• You can do this workout on a treadmill, but I recommend getting outside if weather permits.

• Start with a 5-minute warm-up. That's a slow-to-easy pace to loosen up and warm your muscles.

• Increase your speed, walking as fast as you comfortably can for 60 seconds. Your effort level should be brisk but not so strenuous that you cannot carry on a conversation of short sentences. Slow down if you are too winded to comment on how beautiful the day is. Speed up if you are not breathing hard enough. Bend your arms and swing them to get your upper body into the act to burn more calories. Doing so will also move your legs faster.

• After a minute, slow to a moderate "recovery" pace for 2 minutes. Repeat the sequence five more times plus add a finisher, a 2-minute fast-paced segment before your 5-minute slow-pace cool-down. That's a 30-minute workout.

Take-the-Stairs Interval Workout

■ For a short but intense interval workout that delivers the benefits of a 30-minute exercise session, try stair climbing. Go to the stairwell of your workplace or the bleachers of a local athletic stadium. Walk up the stairs quickly but in control, and walk down at a moderate pace. Repeat. Staircases have roughly a 65 percent grade, which will make climbing harder on your legs and lungs than walking on flat ground. Keep going at this pace for 10 minutes. Make it harder by taking every other stair step going up. Be sure to warm up and cool down.

The Big Burn Walk

On the weekends when you have more time, do a 60-minute walking workout. Choose a scenic route and invite friends along to make it interesting. Walk at a steady pace the entire time. It should be moderately brisk but not as fast as your HIIT walks. You should be able to carry on a normal conversation (long sentences).

Week 2 Challenge

This tweak for your 30-minute HIIT walk is optional, but I recommend trying it. The key to improving fitness is pushing yourself a little more each time.

After a 5-minute easy-pace warm-up, walk as fast as you can for 60 seconds. Then, as you did last week, switch to the moderate-pace recovery segment. This time, however, cut this part of the interval to just 60 seconds. So, you'll be alternating your pace between fast and moderate every 60 seconds. This boosts your exertion level, making your workout more efficient. Don't worry if you can't keep this up for a full 30 minutes. Do as much as you can and then cool down for five minutes. Each time you do this quicker-paced HIIT walk, try to go a bit longer.

Strength-Building Exercise Plan

Stressing your muscles with physical activity regularly is important for good blood sugar control. But there are a lot of other reasons resistance exercise is good for you:

- The more muscle you have on your skeleton, the more calories you burn even when your body is sitting on the couch.

- As you age, your body naturally loses muscle mass. Doing strength exercises slows down the process that replaces lost muscle with fat tissue.

- Preventing muscle loss will help you stay strong enough to maintain independence in your senior years.

- Toned arms and legs look good on you!

  (Don't worry: The type of strength-training workout in this plan will not bulk you up like a superhero.)

For the No Sugar Diet exercise plan, you will do two 15- to 30-minute strength exercise sessions per week. If you haven't done this kind of exercise before, don't sweat it. There's little or nothing to buy. You don't have to go to a gym if you don't want to. You can do everything at home using your own body weight to work your muscles.

Know the Lingo

Warm-up: Just what it sounds like—you warm up your body.

Cool-down: You slow down your effort and bring your heart rate down after a workout.

Repetitions or reps: The number of times you perform a complete exercise.

Sets: The number of times you perform the required repetitions.

Circuit: A round of three or more exercises performed one after another, with little to no rest in between.

Blood-Sugar Burner Body-Weight Circuit

Warm up with a few minutes of total-body movement:

- March in place for a minute, lifting your knees high and swinging your arms.

- Do 20 special jumping jacks, called seal jacks, that are easier on the shoulders for those who have pain there. Stand with feet together and arms across your chest. Jump and spread your legs as in a normal jumping jack but swing your arms out to your sides instead of over your head. Jump your legs back together while simultaneously swinging your arms across your chest. Repeat.

Circuit exercises: Do 8 to 12 repetitions of each of the following exercises. Rest for 30 seconds or less after each exercise. Then go on to the next exercise on the list. The last exercise is called a "finisher." It brings an extra aerobic component to the workout to burn more calories. After completing the finisher, rest for two minutes and then repeat the circuit. During week 2 progress to doing 3 total circuits.

For each body-weight exercise, except for the finisher, I'll give you an easier version and a more challenging version. Choose the one that's right for you and work toward eventually being able to do the more challenging exercise.

Arms-Up Squat

Spread your feet shoulder-width apart with toes pointed slightly outward. Raise both arms above your head. Keeping arms raised, bend your knees and push your butt back as if sitting in a chair. Lower your body until your thighs are parallel with the floor. Pause a second and quickly straighten your legs to stand. Repeat immediately and quickly for 8 to 12 repetitions.

Easier: Do the exercise with your hands on your hips. Don't squat so low. Stop and stand before your thighs are parallel with the floor.

Harder: Do the superhero squat jump. Do the arms-up squat as described above but from the squat position, explosively press your feet into the floor to jump as high as you can so that your feet leave the ground. When your feet touch back down, immediately squat and repeat.

Step Push-Up

Get into a push-up position, but instead of placing your hands on the floor, place them on a stair-step, low bench, or other stable structure that's raised off the floor. Keep your back straight from heels to head. Your arms should be extended straight. Brace your abs. Bend your elbows to lower yourself until your chest is an inch off the step. Pause a second, then push yourself up. Repeat. Do 8 to 12 repetitions.

Easier: Plank. Get on all fours and then extend your legs out straight behind you. Your hands should be directly under your shoulders. Straighten your arms. Brace your core and keep your back flat, forming a straight line from your heels to your head. Hold this rigid position for 30 seconds.

Harder: Standard push-up. Get into a plank position with your palms on the floor directly under your shoulders and your arms straight. Your back should be flat and rigid from your heels to your head. Brace your core. This will help you maintain proper form and burn more calories because you are engaging more muscle fibers. Bend your arms to lower yourself toward the floor until your chest is about an inch from the floor. Press yourself up. Repeat.

Flutter Kick

Lie on your back on the floor with your arms palms-down next to your sides and your toes pointed. Engage your abs to lift your feet about a foot off the floor. Keeping your legs rigid, begin quickly flutter kicking your straight legs back and forth as you would while swimming. Every four kicks equals one rep. Do 8 to 12.

Easier: If your core isn't strong enough to flutter kick, just lift your feet a few inches off the floor, hold for a few seconds, and rest them back on the floor. Repeat.

Harder: Combine a short set of flutter kicks, 5 repetitions, with bicycle crunches, 5 repetitions. This adds rotation and side-bending movements to the core exercise. To do bicycle crunches, lie faceup with your hips and knees bent 90 degrees so that your lower legs are parallel to the floor. Place your fingers on the sides of your forehead. Lift your shoulders off the floor and hold them there. Twist your upper body to the right as you quickly pull your right knee in until it touches your left elbow. Simultaneously straighten your left leg. Return to the starting position and repeat to the left.

Forward Lunge

Stand with your feet together and your hands on your hips. Take a large step forward with your right leg and lower your body toward the floor. Your front leg should bend at the knee, forming a right angle. Your back leg should be bent slightly. Lower yourself until your back knee hovers an inch above the ground and your right thigh is parallel with the floor. Pause in this position for a second.

Press your right foot into the floor to push yourself back to the starting position. Next, step forward with your left foot and repeat. That's one repetition. Do 8 to 12.

Easier: Step forward and lower your body toward the floor. Then rise up to standing but keep your feet in place. Don't step forward but lower yourself again without moving your foot position. Repeat this sequence five times, then switch leg positions and do another five reps without moving your feet.

Harder: Do the forward lunge while holding a dumbbell in each hand to boost resistance. If you don't own dumbbells, hold a jug of water or a large soup can in each hand.

Hip Raise with Press-Out

Lie faceup on the floor or on an exercise mat with your knees bent and your feet flat on the floor. Place your arms out to your sides at 45-degree angles, your palms facing up. Place a 20-inch mini exercise band around your legs above your knees and spread your knees slightly against the resistance as you perform the exercise. Now, raise your hips so that your body forms a straight line from your shoulders to your knees. Pause for up to five seconds in the up position and then lower your body to the starting position. Do 8 to 12.

Easier: Perform the hip raise without doing the press-out part of the exercise using the exercise band. Hold the top position for a second or two while engaging your core and glutes. Do 8 to 12 reps.

Harder: Do the hip raise without the exercise band. But at the top position, when your butt is off the ground, extend one foot out straight while keeping its thigh parallel with the thigh of the other leg. Return your foot to the floor and then repeat with the other leg. After returning that foot to the floor, lower your butt to the floor. Repeat that sequence for 8 to 12 reps.

Mountain Climber Finisher

Remember these fondly from high school? Mountain climbers are a great strength exercise with aerobic benefits to end your circuit. Get into the "up" pushup position with your hands directly under your shoulders and arms straight. Now, rapidly bend and straighten each leg one at a time in alternating fashion. It's like running in place with your hands on the ground. Try bringing your knees to your chest with each pump of your legs. Do these as fast as possible for a full 20 seconds. Then rest and repeat twice more.

DIY PROJECT
Water Weights

Half-gallon or gallon-size water jugs are great for adding resistance to strength-building exercises. Use them as you would a pair of dumbbells. Try them with the farmer's carry, one of the best total-body fat-burning exercises you can do anywhere. Hold a filled water jug in each hand. Stand with your back straight and shoulders pulled back (don't hunch your back). Keeping good posture, walk around your house or yard until you get tired. Put the jugs down, rest for a minute to catch your breath, and then repeat. Work up to doing 6 sets a day.

Appendix A

Unhealthiest Restaurant Meals

These popular menu items may cause the greatest impact on your blood sugar. Make better choices.

WHENEVER YOU EAT outside the home, you lose some control over what you consume. After all, at a restaurant, you're not welcome in the kitchen to see what's going into your meal or how it's being prepared. And even if you could sneak in, the chef probably wouldn't appreciate your suggestions. As you know, restaurant fare is not ideal for people who are trying to reduce consumption of added sugars, lose weight, and prevent type 2 diabetes.

To keep your meal from impacting your health, do some detective work before you head out for dinner. Check the restaurant's website to see if you can find nutrition information for the entrées, and preselect a better choice. The more you know before you go, the easier it will be to avoid carb-and-calorie overload. To that end, here's some useful intel—the worst-offending meals at popular national restaurant chains:

Olive Garden's Eggplant Parmigiana

Nutrition: 1,060 calories, 54 g fat (12 g saturated), 1,190 mg sodium, 113 g carbohydrates, 23 g sugars, 30 g protein, 11 g fiber

Olive Garden is known for its classic unlimited soup, salad, and breadstick lunch duo that starts at $6.99. While this is a dangerous option for people with diabetes—four breadsticks alone are equivalent to 100 grams of carbs—the dinner portion of the Eggplant Parmigiana contains enough carbs to put you into a hyperglycemic state immediately after consumption.

Eat This Instead! **Chicken Margherita**

Chili's Crispy Honey & Chipotle Waffles

Nutrition: 2,450 calories, 123 g fat (39 g saturated), 5,720 mg sodium, 276 g carbohydrates, 113 g sugars, 61 g protein, 11 g fiber

Can we agree that this chicken and waffle rendition constitutes one of the worst high-carb meals on the planet at 276 grams? What's even worse is the sugar content. To give you perspective, 113 grams is equivalent to 28¼ teaspoons of table sugar. You would consume this much added sugar by eating 14 Reese's Peanut Butter Cups.

Eat This Instead! **6-ounce Sirloin with Grilled Avocado**

Applebee's Classic Combo

Nutrition: 2,270 calories, 131 g fat (41 g saturated), 7,240 mg sodium, 192 g carbohydrates, 13 g sugars, 83 g protein, 16 g fiber

The Classic Combo with fried mozzarella sticks, fatty spinach and artichoke dip, cheese chicken quesadillas, and fried wings is a diabetes disaster. Just look at its carb and calorie counts. It's also too high in protein to be healthy for people with blood sugar issues. Check with your doctor to see how much protein is adequate for your body.

Eat This Instead! **Green Goddess Wedge Salad**

Cracker Barrel's Buttermilk Pancakes with Fruit Topping

Nutrition: Pancakes alone: 630 calories, 16 g fat (3 g saturated), 2,640 mg sodium, 11 g carbohydrates, 9 g sugars, 9 g protein, 2 g fiber

When you add any one of the three fruit toppings—country peach, sweet ripe blackberry, and cinnamon spiced apple—paired with whipped cream, you're eating up to 380 additional calories, 75 grams of carbs, and 68 grams of sugar. Opt out of this carb-heavy disaster and order a bowl of oatmeal topped with fresh fruit to get your sweet fix.

Eat This Instead! **Apple 'N' Cinnamon Oatmeal**

TGI Friday's Jack Daniel's® Ribs: Full-Rack with Coleslaw & Seasoned Fries

Nutrition: 1,600 calories, 73 g fat (25 g saturated), 2,860 mg sodium, 73 g carbohydrates, 126 g sugars, 69 g protein, 7 g fiber

The American Heart Association recommends that you consume no more than 25 grams of added sugar a day for optimal health. This full rack of ribs has a little over five times that amount.

Eat This Instead! **Lunch portion of the Strawberry Fields Salad with Grilled Chicken with Balsamic Vinaigrette**

Red Lobster's Shrimp Linguini Alfredo

Nutrition: 1,340 calories, 59 g fat (24 g saturated fat), 2,410 mg sodium, 118 g carbohydrates, 5 g sugars, 80 g protein, 8 g fiber

The full-size portion of this meal is another dangerously high-in-protein selection. With this shrimp and pasta dish, you're exceeding your protein limit...and in a single sitting!

Eat This Instead! **Lighthouse Snow Crab Legs**

California Pizza Kitchen's Thai Chicken Pizza

Nutrition: 1,290 calories, 45 g fat (15 g saturated), 3,190 mg sodium, 167 g carbohydrates, 27 g sugars, 63 g protein, 10 g fiber

California Pizza Kitchen (CPK) may offer some delicious pizza, but that carb content is just way too high for a person with diabetes or someone trying to avoid blood sugar problems. Tip: Women should try to keep carbs to under 60 grams per meal. Men should avoid foods over 75 grams. This pizza alone takes care of your carb allowances for lunch and dinner, and then some.

Eat This Instead! **Shaved Mushroom + Spinach Flatbread**

Carrabba's Rigatoni Campagnolo with Gluten-Free Pasta

Nutrition: 1,210 calories, 45 g fat (18 g saturated), 6,730 mg sodium, 158 g carbohydrates, 19 g sugars, 52 g protein, 19 g fiber

Believe it or not, gluten-free doesn't always mean the dish is healthier. In fact, the gluten-free variety of this dish has 44 more grams of carbs than the variety with whole-grain spaghetti.

Eat This Instead! **½ portion of the Parmesan-crusted Chicken Arugula with a side of steamed spinach**

Buffalo Wild Wings' Boneless Asian Zing

Nutrition: 1,710 calories, 74 g fat (29 g saturated), 5,330 mg sodium, 184 g carbohydrates, 12 g fiber, 62 g sugars, 77 g protein

Talk about a carb, sugar, and protein overload! The nutrition information listed above is indicative of the large portion size. It would be better to order the small size, but even that has 101 grams of carbs, 40 grams of sugar, and 39 grams of protein.

Eat This Instead! **Up to five single wings (boneless or traditional) of any flavor**

PF Chang's Chicken Pad Thai

Nutrition: 1,120 calories, 22 g fat (4 g saturated), 4,970 mg sodium, 166 g carbohydrates, 50 g sugars, 52 g protein, 9 g fiber

Chicken Pad Thai made anywhere has high carb and sugar numbers, but stay away from this PF Chang's version for another big reason: nearly 5,000 mg of sodium, more than double what the CDC recommends for people under age 50 per day and triple the recommended 1,500 for those over 50.

Eat This Instead! **Handmade Shrimp Dumplings (steamed)**

Red Robin's Nacho Chicken Bacon Wrap

Nutrition: 1,480 calories, 81 g fat (26 g saturated), 3,080 mg sodium, 127 g carbohydrates, 4 g sugars, 54 g protein, 18 g fiber

On the bright side, this wrap has a relatively low sugar content. But calories, carbs, and sodium are too high. Plus, if you order it with one of the restaurant's iconic shakes, you'll add 162 grams of carbs and 141 grams of sugar.

Eat This Instead! **Ensenada Chicken Platter**

Texas Roadhouse's Fish and Chips

Nutrition: 1,160 calories, 48 g fat (9 g saturated), 6,120 mg sodium, 122 g carbohydrates, 4 g sugars, 59 g protein, 6 g fiber

The batter on the cod and the steak fries turn this fish dish into a high-carb, ultra-high-sodium nightmare. Note that the nutrition facts don't account for the tartar sauce on the side. That adds 390 calories, 38 g fat, 530 mg of sodium, 14 g carbs, and 9 g sugars.

Eat This Instead! **Grilled BBQ Chicken**

Bob Evans' Biscuit Breaded Fried Shrimp

Nutrition: 1,520 calories, 86 g fat (33 g saturated), 3,850 mg sodium, 155 g carbohydrates, 35 g sugars, 36 g protein, 10 g fiber

Here's a good example of why you should never bread and deep-fry shrimp. Or serve biscuits with an already breaded meal.

Eat This Instead! **Grilled Salmon Fillet—Fit from the Farm variety**

Appendix B

Glycemic Load Chart

The glycemic load (GL) of common foods expressed as the percentage of the GL of a slice of white bread

USE A SINGLE SLICE of white bread as a comparison guide for understanding the glycemic load (impact of a food on raising blood sugar) of various foods.

White Bread / 1 slice / Glycemic Load=100

Food Item	Description	Typical Serving	Glycemic Load
BAKED GOODS			
Oatmeal cookie	1 medium	1 oz	102
Apple muffin, sugarless	2½" diameter	2½ oz	107
Cookie, average, all types	1 medium	1 oz	114
Croissant	1 medium	1½ oz	127
Crumpet	1 medium	2 oz	148
Bran muffin	2½" diameter	2 oz	149

Food Item	Description	Typical Serving	Glycemic Load
Pastry	Average serving	2 oz	149
Chocolate cake	1 slice (4"x4"x1")	3 oz	154
Vanilla wafers	4 wafers	1 oz	159
Graham cracker	1 rectangle	1 oz	159
Blueberry muffin	2½" diameter	2 oz	169
Carrot cake	1 square (3"x3"x1½")	2 oz	199
Carrot muffin	2½" diameter	2 oz	199
Waffle	7" diameter	2½ oz	203
Doughnut	1 medium	2 oz	205
Cupcake	2½" diameter	1½ oz	213
Angel food cake	1 slice (4"x4"x1")	2 oz	216
English muffin	1 medium	2 oz	224
Pound cake	1 slice (4"x4"x1")	3 oz	241
Corn muffin	2½" diameter	2 oz	299
Pancake	5" diameter	2½ oz	346

BREADS AND ROLLS

Food Item	Description	Typical Serving	Glycemic Load
Tortilla (wheat)	1 medium	1⅜ oz	64
Pizza crust	1 slice	3½ oz	70
Tortilla (corn)	1 medium	1 ¼ oz	87
White bread	½" slice	1 oz	100
Whole-meal rye bread	⅜" slice	2 oz	114
Sourdough bread	⅜" slice	1½ oz	114
Oat bran bread	⅜" slice	1½ oz	128
Whole-wheat bread	½" slice	1½ oz	129

Food Item	Description	Typical Serving	Glycemic Load
Rye bread	⅜" slice	1½ oz	142
Banana bread, sugarless	1 slice (4"x4"x1")	3 oz	170
80% whole-kernel oat bread	⅜" slice	1½ oz	170
Buckwheat Bread	⅜" slice	1½ oz	183
80% whole-kernel barley bread	⅜" slice	1½ oz	185
Pita	8" diameter	2 oz	189
Hamburger bun	Top and bottom, 5" diameter	2½ oz	213
80% whole-kernel wheat bread	⅜" slice	2¼ oz	213
French bread	½ slice	2 oz	284
Bagel	1 medium	3⅓ oz	340

BREAKFAST CEREALS

All-Bran	½ cup	1 oz	85
Muesli	1 cup	1 oz	95
Oatmeal	1 cup	8 oz	123
Special K	1 cup	1 oz	133
Cheerios	1 cup	1 oz	142
Shredded Wheat	1 cup	1 oz	142
Grape-Nuts	1 cup	1 oz	142
Granola	1 cup	1 oz	142
Puffed wheat	1 cup	1 oz	151
Kashi	1 cup	1 oz	151
Instant oatmeal	1 cup	8 oz	154
Cream of Wheat, cooked	1 cup	8 oz	154

Food Item	Description	Typical Serving	Glycemic Load
Total	1 cup	1 oz	161
Froot Loops	1 cup	1 oz	170
Cornflakes	1 cup	1 oz	199
Rice Krispies	1 cup	1 oz	208
Rice Chex	1 cup	1 oz	218
Raisin Bran	1 cup	2 oz	227

CANDY AND SNACKS

Food Item	Description	Typical Serving	Glycemic Load
Sugar-free milk chocolate	2 squares (1"x1"x ¼")	1 oz	17
Life Savers	1 piece	⅒ oz	20
Peanut M&M'S	1 snack-size package	¾ oz	43
Dark chocolate	2 squares (1"x1"x ¼")	1 oz	44
Licorice	1 twist	⅓ oz	45
White chocolate	2 squares (1"x1"x ¼")	⅔ oz	49
Milk chocolate	2 squares (1"x1"x ¼")	1 oz	68
Jelly beans	6 beans	½ oz	104
Granola bar, **apple or cranberry**	1 bar	1 oz	131
Snickers bar	1 regular-size bar	2 oz	218

CHIPS AND CRACKERS

Food Item	Description	Typical Serving	Glycemic Load
Potato chips	Small bag	1 oz	62
Corn chips	1 package	1 oz	97
Popcorn	4 cups	1 oz	114

Food Item	Description	Typical Serving	Glycemic Load
Rye crisp	1 rectangle	1 oz	125
Wheat Thins	4 small	1 oz	136
Soda crackers	2 regular size	1 oz	136
Pretzels	Small bag	1 oz	151
Rice cakes	3 regular size	1 oz	190

DAIRY PRODUCTS

Food Item	Description	Typical Serving	Glycemic Load
Cheese	2"x2"x1" slice	2 oz	<15
Butter	1 Tbsp	¼ oz	<15
Margarine	Typical serving	¼ oz	<15
Sour cream	Typical serving	2 oz	<15
Yogurt, full-fat **(unsweetened)**	½ cup	4 oz	17
Milk (whole)	8 oz glass	8 oz	37
Milk (fat-free)	8 oz glass	8 oz	41
Yogurt, low-fat **(sweetened)**	½ cup	4 oz	57
Soy milk	8 oz glass	8 oz	62
Vanilla ice cream **(high fat)**	½ cup	4 oz	68
Chocolate milk (low-fat)	8 oz glass	8 oz	82
Custard	½ cup	4½ oz	89
Chocolate pudding	½ cup	4½ oz	89
Chocolate ice cream **(high-fat)**	½ cup	4½ oz	91
Vanilla ice cream (low-fat)	½ cup	4 oz	159
Frozen tofu	½ cup	4 oz	379

Food Item	Description	Typical Serving	Glycemic Load
FRUIT			
Strawberries	1 cup	5½ oz	13
Apricot	1 medium	2 oz	24
Grapefruit	1 half	4½ oz	32
Plum	1 medium	3 oz	36
Nectarine	1 medium	4 oz	38
Cherries, dark	8	2 oz	43
Kiwifruit	1 medium	3 oz	43
Peaches, **canned in natural juice**	½ cup	4 oz	45
Peaches, fresh	1 medium	4 oz	47
Grapes	½ cup	2½ oz	47
Pineapple	1 slice (¾"x 3½" wide)	3 oz	50
Watermelon	1 cup cubed	5½ oz	52
Cantaloupe	1 cup cubed	5½ oz	52
Pear	1 medium	6 oz	57
Mango	½ cup	3 oz	57
Orange	1 medium	6 oz	71
Apricot, dried	½ cup	2 oz	76
Apple	1 medium	5½ oz	78
Banana	1 medium	3¼ oz	85
Prunes, pitted, dried	½ cup	2 oz	104
Peaches, **canned in heavy syrup**	½ cup	4 oz	112
Raisins	2 Tbsp	1 oz	133

Food Item	Description	Typical Serving	Glycemic Load
Figs	3 medium	2 oz	151
Dates	5 medium	1½ oz	298

MEATS, FISH AND EGGS

Food Item	Description	Typical Serving	Glycemic Load
Beef	10-oz steak	10 oz	<15
Pork	Two 5-oz chops	10 oz	<15
Chicken	1 breast	10 oz	<15
Fish	8-oz fillet	8 oz	<15
Lamb	Three 4-oz chops	12 oz	<15
Eggs	1 large	1½ oz	<15

RESTAURANT FOODS

Food Item	Description	Typical Serving	Glycemic Load
Deluxe burger, no bun	1 medium	3¼ oz	<15
Pizza, outer rim of crust	1 slice	3 oz	45
Wheat tortilla, bean filled	1 burrito	4 oz	50
Chicken nuggets	4 oz	4 oz	70
Deluxe burger, **minus top bun**	1 medium	4¼ oz	80
Cannelloni, **spinach, ricotta**	2 tubes	12 oz	88
Pizza, crust intact	1 slice	4 oz	90
French fries	Medium serving (McDonald's)	5¼ oz	219
Chili con carne	1 cup	8 oz	91
Veggie burger	1 medium	3½ oz	140
Deluxe hamburger	1 medium	5¾ oz	170
Fish sandwich	1 medium	4½ oz	200

Food Item	Description	Typical Serving	Glycemic Load
Chicken korma and rice	10 oz	10 oz	210
Chicken sandwich	1 medium	6½ oz	260

NUTS

Food Item	Description	Typical Serving	Glycemic Load
Peanuts	¼ cup	1¼ oz	<15
Walnuts	¼ cup	1¼ oz	<15
Almonds	¼ cup	1¼ oz	<15
Cashews	¼ cup	1¼ oz	21

PASTA

Food Item	Description	Typical Serving	Glycemic Load
Asian bean noodles	1 cup	5 oz	118
Spaghetti, whole grain	1 cup	5 oz	126
Vermicelli	1 cup	5 oz	126
Spaghetti (boiled 5 min.)	1 cup	5 oz	142
Fettuccine	1 cup	5 oz	142
Noodles (instant, boiled 2 min.)	1 cup	5 oz	150
Capellini	1 cup	5 oz	158
Spaghetti (boiled 10 to 15 min.)	1 cup	5 oz	166
Linguine	1 cup	5 oz	181
Macaroni	1 cup	5 oz	181
Rice noodles	1 cup	5 oz	181
Spaghetti (boiled 20 min.)	1 cup	5 oz	213
Macaroni and cheese (boxed)	1 cup	5 oz	252
Gnocchi	1 cup	5 oz	260

Food Item	Description	Typical Serving	Glycemic Load
SOUPS			
Tomato soup	1 cup	8 oz	55
Minestrone	1 cup	8 oz	64
Lentil soup	1 cup	8 oz	82
Split-pea soup	1 cup	8 oz	145
Black bean soup	1 cup	8 oz	154
SWEETENERS			
Agave	2 tsp	1¼ oz	<15
Artificial sweeteners	1 tsp	⅙ oz	<15
Honey	1 tsp	⅙ oz	16
Table sugar	1 rounded tsp	⅙ oz	28
Syrup	¼ cup	2 oz	364
VEGETABLES AND LEGUMES			
Carrots, raw	1 medium (7½")	3 oz	11
Lettuce	1 cup	2½ oz	<15
Spinach	1 cup	2½ oz	<15
Cucumber	1 cup	6½ oz	<15
Mushrooms	½ cup	2½ oz	<15
Asparagus	4 spears	3 oz	<15
Bell Peppers	½ medium	2 oz	<15
Broccoli	½ cup	1½ oz	<15
Chickpeas, boiled	2 Tbsp	1 oz	<15
Tomato	1 medium	5 oz	<15
Peas	¼ cup	1½ oz	16
Carrots, boiled	⅔ cup	3 oz	21

Food Item	Description	Typical Serving	Glycemic Load
Fava beans	½ cup	3 oz	32
Lentils	½ cup	3½ cups	33
Butter beans	½ cup	3 oz	34
Cannellini beans	½ cup	3 oz	34
Kidney beans	½ cup	3 oz	40
Navy beans	½ cup	3 oz	40
Parsnips	½ cup	3 oz	50
Lima beans	½ cup	3 oz	57
Refried pinto beans	½ cup	3 oz	57
Black-eyed peas	½ cup	3 oz	74
Yam	½ cup	5 oz	123

GRAINS

Food Item	Description	Typical Serving	Glycemic Load
Quinoa	1 cup	6½ oz	160
Potato, instant mashed	¾ cup	5 oz	161
Sweet potato	½ cup	5 oz	161
Corn on the cob	1 ear	5⅓ oz	171
Couscous	½ cup	4 oz	174
Brown and wild rice mix	1 cup	6½ oz	221
Brown rice	1 cup	6½ oz	222
Baked potato	1 medium	5 oz	264
Basmati rice	1 cup	6½ oz	271
White rice	1 cup	6½ oz	283
Sticky white rice	1 cup	6½ oz	295

Food Item	Description	Typical Serving	Glycemic Load
ALCOHOLIC BEVERAGES			
Spirits	1½ oz	1½ oz	<15
Red wine	6-oz glass	6 oz	<15
White wine	6-oz glass	6 oz	<15
Beer	12-oz can/bottle	12 oz	70
NONALCOHOLIC BEVERAGES			
Tomato juice	6-oz glass	6 oz	27
V8 juice	6-oz glass	6 oz	27
Carrot juice	6-oz glass	6 oz	68
Grapefruit juice, **unsweetened**	6-oz glass	6 oz	75
Apple juice, unsweetened	6-oz glass	6 oz	82
Chocolate milk	8-oz glass	8 oz	82
Orange juice	6-oz glass	6 oz	89
Prune juice	6-oz glass	6 oz	102
Cranberry juice	6-oz glass	6 oz	209
Pineapple juice, **unsweetened**	6-oz glass	6 oz	109
Raspberry smoothie	8-oz glass	8 oz	127
Lemonade	8-oz glass	8 oz	136
Ensure	8-oz glass	8 oz	182
Coca-Cola	12-oz can	12 oz	218
Gatorade	20-oz bottle	20 oz	273
Orange soda	12-oz glass	12 oz	314